PRAISE FROM THE MEDICAL COMMUNITY FOR "THE MEDICAL MANUAL FOR RELIGIO-CULTURAL COMPETENCE"

"*The Medical Manual* represents an exciting step forward in how we prepare today's health care professionals for effectively treating and interacting with patients of all religious backgrounds. ... [It] will serve as an indispensable resource for all providers."

Wayne E. Keathley
President and Chief Operating Officer, Mount Sinai Medical Center

"*The Medical Manual* is an excellent source of information for nurses, who are often instrumental in helping patients get their religious needs met."

Deloras Jones, RN, MS
President and Executive Director, California Institute for Nursing & Health Care

"Tanenbaum's *Medical Manual* is a valuable and comprehensive resource that will help physicians, nurses, chaplains and other health and human service professionals to provide care, which is more sensitive and responsive to the needs of our increasingly diverse population. ... I'm pleased to highly recommend this excellent new resource to clinicians, educators and administrators who are interested in the real bottom line: 'To cure sometimes, to care often, to comfort always.'"

Robert C. Like, MD, MS
Professor and Director,
Center for Healthy Families and Cultural Diversity
Department of Family Medicine, UMDNJ-Robert Wood Johnson Medical School

"Tanenbaum's new resource, *The Medical Manual*, is a concise yet comprehensive resource that sensitively provides information about religious traditions, beliefs and practices. The understanding one gains with each chapter will assist occupational therapists to work more meaningfully with patients and their families. I want all of my students to read this book!"

Janet Falk-Kessler, Ed.D., OTR, FAOTA
Director, Programs in Occupational Therapy
Columbia University

"Tanenbaum's text, *The Medical Manual*, enhances the provider-patient relationship by helping the entire team of health care providers (neurologists, physiatrists, psychiatrists, occupational therapists, physical therapists, speech-language pathologists and social workers) incorporate religious sensitivity into their treatment plan. By respectfully addressing religion — an area that is often a key part of people's identities — providers will help Parkinson patients enhance their quality of life and more effectively manage their disease."

Ruth Hagestuen, RN, MA
Director, NYU Parkinson and Movement Disorder Center
A National Parkinson Foundation Center of Excellence
NYU Langone Medical Center, Center of Excellence on Brain Aging

The Medical Manual for Religio-Cultural Competence

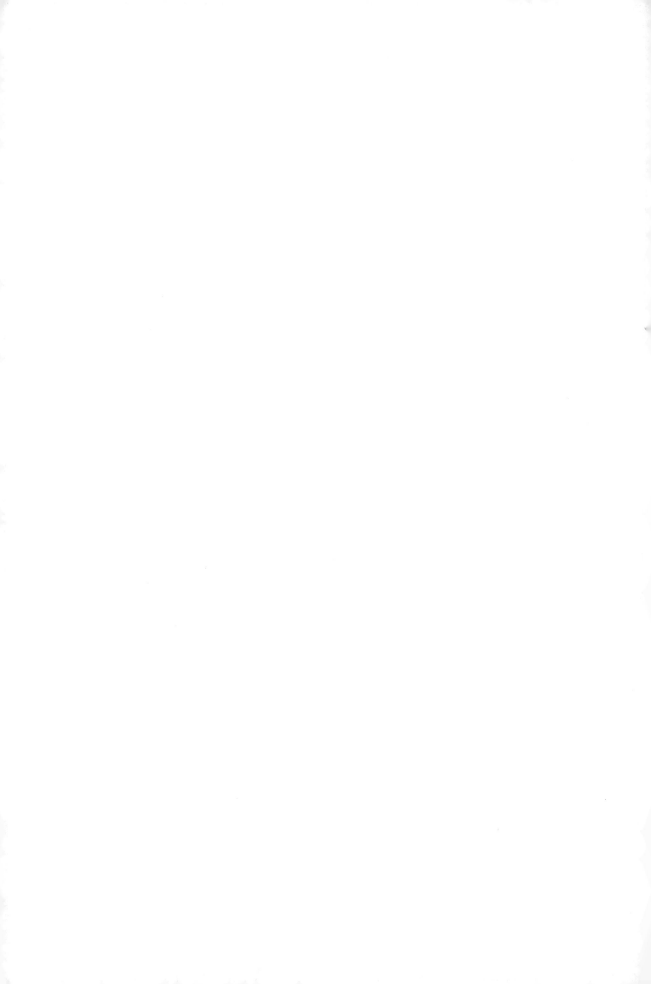

The Medical Manual for Religio-Cultural Competence

••••

Caring for Religiously Diverse Populations

••••

TANENBAUM / CENTER FOR INTERRELIGIOUS UNDERSTANDING

© 2009, TANENBAUM/Center for Interreligious Understanding.

This publication is in copyright, with all rights reserved. No part of this book may be used or reproduced, stored in a retrieval system, or transmitted in any other form or by any other means, electronic, mechanical, photocopying, recording or otherwise without the express written permission of TANENBAUM/Center for Interreligious Understanding.

First published 2009.

TANENBAUM/Center for Interreligious Understanding has no responsibility for the persistence or accuracy of URLs for external or third-party Internet Web sites referred to in this publication and does not guarantee that any content on such Web sites is, or will remain, accurate or appropriate.

For other information contact TANENBAUM/Center for Interreligious Understanding
254 W. 31st St, 7th floor, New York, NY 10001

For permissions to use or reproduce or to purchase additional copies, contact TANENBAUM/Center for Interreligious Understanding at healthcare@tanenbaum.org or visit www.tanenbaum.org.

First edition sponsored by EmblemHealth, Inc., www.emblemhealth.com.

*"There are many reasons why
health care professionals need to assess
and address the religious and spiritual needs
of patients and cannot leave this entirely
up to chaplains and other clergy.
The patient is a unique person
with physical, psychological, social and
spiritual needs that must be addressed
if health care is to be maximized
and the whole person treated."*

— Harold G. Koenig, M.D.

ACKNOWLEDGEMENTS

....

Any project of this magnitude takes many moving parts to create. Tanenbaum is deeply grateful for the support of many uncommonly dedicated and talented people in the production of *The Medical Manual for Religio-Cultural Competence*.

Tanenbaum is indebted to Georgette F. Bennett, our President and Founder, who first conceived of the contribution that Tanenbaum could make to the field of religious diversity in health care.

We were also privileged to have been guided by advisory bodies of scholars, practitioners and others who gave freely of their time and energy and provided thought-provoking feedback. Thank you to Dr. Herbert Benson, Harvard Medical School; Dr. John Bucchino, Our Lady of Peace Church, Brooklyn, New York; Dr. John S. Caskey, Internal and Integrative Medicine, Santa Fe, New Mexico; Dr. Alessandro Di Rocco, Chair of Neurology at NYU Medical Center; Dr. Harold Koenig, Duke University; Dr. David Muller, Dean of Medical Education at the Mt. Sinai School of Medicine; Dr. Christina Puchalski, George Washington University; and John White, Souci Grimsley and Karen Chaikin of EmblemHealth, Inc.

The chapters on individual religious traditions would not have been possible without the critiques of our expert reviewers: George Handzo of the HealthCare Chaplaincy; Rabbi Charles Sheer of the Center for Jewish Studies in Pastoral Care; Professor Francis X. Clooney of Harvard Divinity School; Imam Shamsi Ali of the 96th Street Mosque; Dr. Susan Cameron of the Santa Fe Indian Hospital; Vivienne Lo and Michael Stanley-Baker of the Wellcome Trust Centre for the History of Medicine at University College London; Dr. George Brandon of the Sophie Davis School of Biomedical Education at the City University of New York; and Dr. Craig Gerard-Francois Centrie of the University of Buffalo. Thanks also to the Zen Hospice Project, the Sikh Coalition, and the International Shintō Federation for their assistance.

We owe particular thanks to Tanenbaum staff past and present, whose tireless work was critical in bringing *The Medical Manual* to life. First, we extend profound thanks to Michelle Weber, who was pivotal in its conception, spearheaded the project and worked with colleague Rebekah Walter to research, write and push the manual to completion. Without their committed efforts, this manual would not exist.

We extend our appreciation to Rachel Maryles, Luke Bergamini and Charmaine Chua for jumping in whenever additional hands were needed, from fact-checking to proofreading. We also acknowledge former colleagues Rachel Ehrlich, part of the original conversations about the manual, and Laura Votey for her dedication to its completion.

All of us also gratefully acknowledge the work of Ron Albrecht and Benjamin Gaunt for making *The Medical Manual* look as good as it reads.

And finally, we thank our Executive Vice President & CEO, Joyce S. Dubensky, whose leadership, belief in the power of this manual to improve health care and commitment to excellence inspired us all.

Table of Contents

Introduction by Joyce S. Dubensky, Executive Vice President & CEO ... i

How to Use the Medical Manual ... iii

PART ONE
An Introduction to Religion & Health Care ... 1
    1. What Patients Want, What Doctors Are Doing ... 2
    2. Talking About Religion: Challenges and Opportunities ... 5
    3. Addressing Religion in Care: Good Business Sense ... 7
    4. Demographic Changes and Their Impact ... 9
    5. Not Just Religion: Spirituality and Patient Care ... 11

PART TWO
How to Understand Your Patients ... 15
    1. Spiritual Assessment Instruments ... 16
    2. Understanding Your Patients: Communication Skills ... 21
    3. When Religion Becomes Relevant: Spiritual Journeys ... 23
    4. Incorporating Spiritual Assessments into Treatment Plans ... 27
    5. Checklists and Organizational Tools ... 28

PART THREE
Religions of the World & Their Applications to Health Care ... 43
    1. Judaism ... 44
        Overview FAQ ... 44
        Intersections with Health Care: FAQ ... 47
        Judaism: Intersections with Health Care ... 51
        For More Reading ... 59

    2. Christianity ... 60
        Overview FAQ ... 60
        Intersections with Health Care: FAQ ... 64
        Christianity: Intersections with Health Care ... 67
        For More Reading ... 77

3. Islam — **78**
    Overview FAQ — 78
    Intersections with Health Care: FAQ — 81
    Islam: Intersections with Health Care — 85
    For More Reading — 95

4. Buddhism — **96**
    Overview FAQ — 96
    Intersections with Health Care: FAQ — 99
    Buddhism: Intersections with Health Care — 101
    For More Reading — 107

5. Hinduism — **108**
    Overview FAQ — 108
    Intersections with Health Care: FAQ — 110
    Hinduism: Intersections with Health Care — 114
    For More Reading — 122

6. Sikhism — **123**
    Overview FAQ — 123
    Intersections with Health Care: FAQ — 125
    Sikhism: Intersections with Health Care — 128
    For More Reading — 137

7. Shintō — **137**
    Overview FAQ — 137
    Intersections with Health Care: FAQ — 139
    Shintō: Intersections with Health Care — 141
    For More Reading — 147

8. Traditional Chinese — **148**
    Overview FAQ — 148
    Intersections with Health Care: FAQ — 152
    Traditional Chinese: Intersections with Health Care — 156
    For More Reading — 163

9. American Indian & Alaska Natives (AIAN) — **164**
    Overview FAQ — 164
    Intersections with Health Care: FAQ — 166
    AIAN: Intersections with Health Care — 169
    For More Reading — 176

10. Afro-Caribbean Traditions — **177**
    Overview FAQ — 177
    Intersections with Health Care: FAQ — 180
    Afro-Caribbean Traditions: Intersections with Health Care — 183
    For More Reading — 190

PART FOUR
Practitioners' Responsibilities — **192**
    1. Practitioners' Responsibilities — 193
    2. Six Steps to a Religiously Inclusive Practice — 195
    3. Organizational Resources — 198

PART FIVE
Key Interventions — **200**
    1. Setting Boundaries: Proselytizing & Inappropriate Religious Expression in a Health Care Setting — 201
    2. Working with Family, Friends and Other Caregivers — 204
    3. Working Effectively with Chaplains — 207
    4. Pastoral Care Resources — 210
    5. Navigating the December Dilemma — 211
    6. Overcoming Barriers to Care — 214

ADDENDUM
Checklists, Tools and Organizational Resources — **218**
    1. Setting Boundaries — 220
    2. Navigating the December Dilemma — 221
        — Checklist — 221
        — Five to Know — 222
    3. Working with Family, Friends and Other Caregivers — 223
        — Tracking Sheet — 224
    4. Pastoral Care: Organizational Resources — 225
        — Chaplain & Clergy Contact Sheet — 226
    5. Special Community Needs: Organizational Resources — 227
        — Tracking Sheet — 228

A LETTER FROM JOYCE S. DUBENSKY, EXECUTIVE VICE PRESIDENT AND CEO, TANENBAUM

• • • •

The book you're holding represents three years of development, research and writing. It reflects countless hours of work by Tanenbaum's talented staff and the assistance of dozens of experts.

More importantly, *The Medical Manual* represents a promise. It is a strategic roadmap to fundamental shifts in the practice of medicine toward more responsive, patient-centered care. Whether you are a physician, nurse, physical or occupational therapist, social worker, home health worker – anyone who comes into direct contact with a patient – this book will help improve your interactions with those in need of your care and services.

We live in a religious world. Globally and in the U.S., over 4/5 of people identify as religious. For many, religion influences countless day to day decisions: What to wear. What to eat. How we handle stress. Who we interact with, and how.

These are the decisions that affect how many of us live our lives – and the ways we access health care (or don't). We may choose not to have elective surgery on a holy day. We may insist on critical dietary restrictions, or persist in our traditional diet even though it worsens our health. We may choose traditional herbal therapies, or may integrate them with Western-style medicine. We may tell our doctors about these alternative therapies or keep quiet. We may have important religious practices around reproductive and sexual health, birth, hospitalization, surgery or end of life.

But too often, we have providers who don't know about or understand our needs. This book – *The Medical Manual* – is the resource that can change all that.

Religio-cultural competence is no longer an "extra" or "soft" topic. It is a necessity for providers committed to providing high-quality care. The manual is a comprehensive resource that can help all health providers understand how religion interacts with healthcare, and why patients make the decisions they do. This will create stronger provider-patient relationships and ultimately better health outcomes.

Tanenbaum has trained hundreds of health care practitioners from around the world to better understand how religious beliefs and practices affect patient care. Now, *The Medical Manual for Religio-Cultural Competence* extends our training, supporting those we have trained and acting as a resource for those we have not.

We hope that *The Medical Manual* will become a critical part of your practice. We know it can change your patients' lives – and your own. And when it does, the promise of *The Medical Manual* will become a lived reality.

Joyce S. Dubensky

HOW TO USE THE MEDICAL MANUAL FOR RELIGIO-CULTURAL COMPETENCE

• • • •

Welcome to The Medical Manual for Religio-Cultural Competence. By accessing this resource, you're demonstrating a desire to understand and connect with your patients as whole people: Congratulations!

This manual has been designed to get you the basic information you need on religious issues quickly *and* to provide more in-depth explanations for those times when you need to know more.

The five sections of this resource cover the gamut, from the business case for becoming religiously competent to end-of-life practices of Afro-Caribbean religious traditions, to guidelines to dealing with proselytizing in the health care workplace. In each of the sections and sub-sections, you'll find a range of materials:

- The **Chapters** contain the core information on their topics.
- **FAQs** provide quick answers when you need information *now*.
- **Resources** guide you to other valuable readings.
- **Organizational Resources** are tools you can photocopy and use to self-assess, organize information, and plot the integration of religion into patients' treatment plans.

Jump to a FAQ when you need to know basic information fast: What are kosher dietary restrictions? Try page 48. What should be done with a Sikh's religious items if they need to be removed for treatment? Jump to page 125. How should a Buddhist's body be handled after death? Head to page 101.

Use the main text when you have more time or need to understand the justification behind a particular practice: Why won't a Native American patient consent to treatment without the agreement of a grandparent? Why won't a Jehovah's Witness accept a transfusion?

There are caveats as well. While this manual is a tool to help you understand and meet patients' religious needs, it should *not* be read as suggesting that religion necessarily enhances patient care, or that practitioners are free to discuss their own religious beliefs with patients. Rather, this resource will help you improve the religio-cultural competence of the care you offer to patients for whom religion is *already* an issue.

Pick a section and get started!

- Part I: An Introduction to Religion & Health Care
- Part II: How to Understand Your Patients
- Part III: Religions of the World & Their Applications to Health Care
- Part IV: Practitioners' Responsibilities
- Part V: Key Interventions

PART I

••••

An Introduction to Religion & Health Care

••••

What Patients Want, What Doctors Are Doing

Talking About Religion: Challenges and Opportunities

Addressing Religion in Care: Good Business Sense

Demographic Changes and Their Impact

Not Just Religion: Spirituality and Patient Care

PART 1: AN INTRODUCTION TO RELIGION & HEALTH CARE

1

What Patients Want, What Doctors are Doing

What do patients want from their physicians and other health care providers?

Most people have a fairly clear set of expectations for practitioners. At a minimum, patients expect providers to be skilled professionals who know how to ask all the right questions so that they can fully treat the patient. They expect that a doctor or nurse will ask about their medical history, drinking and smoking habits, or medication. They expect that other providers will ask questions pertinent to their specialties. Increasingly, they also expect the practitioner to inquire about their religious beliefs and know what to do with the information once they get it.

Patients' expectations of providers shift over time. Fifty years ago, patients may not have expected a physician to ask a single woman about contraceptive use. Twenty-five years ago, they might not have expected questions about mental well-being or antidepressant use. Ten years ago, a patient may have had to bring a family member to the hospital to translate for him/her if s/he had limited English proficiency.

Much of that has now changed. Today, practitioners routinely ask about sexual activity and emotional health. And as cultural competence and language access become more widely accepted as core clinical competencies for health care providers, many facilities provide translation services for a range of languages and have begun encouraging providers to be mindful of cultural differences (for example, around communication norms or body language) in patient interactions.

Today, many people also want—and expect—that health care practitioners will inquire into their religious backgrounds. Religion is one of the largest components of culture, if not *the* largest, and a substantial part of many people's personal identity. In addition, America is a highly religious society; 92% of the people in the United States believe in a higher power and, for many, this means more than just church at Christmas. Around 80% of people say that religion is "very" or "somewhat" important in their lives. This is especially important for health care providers because religion often directly impacts health care; 41% of people say that religion directly influenced a health care decision they made for themselves or for a loved one.

In light of that, it's not surprising that patients want their health care practitioners to ask about religion; 83% of people report that they would like their physicians to ask in at least some circumstances:

- A full 20% of people *always* want their providers to ask about religion, even during routine doctor visits.

- The remaining 63% want their practitioners to ask in particular circumstances, especially:

    - End of life;
    - Diagnosis of a serious medical condition;
    - Death of a loved one;
    - On admission to the hospital; and
    - While taking a medical history during an initial doctor's visit.

- Only 17% of people *never* wanted to be asked.

Patients have a wide variety of reasons for wanting the question to be asked, some related to trust and others to actual medical outcomes. The most commonly reported reasons they want their providers to understand their religious beliefs include[1]:

- So the doctor can understand how a patient's beliefs influence how s/he deals with sickness;

- To deepen physician-patient understanding;

- So the doctor can give more accurate medical advice;

- So the doctor can better advise a patient how to take care of himself/herself; and

- Because a doctor might change medical treatment.

In addition, patients—even patients with no religious affiliation—have greater trust in practitioners who ask about their religious or spiritual backgrounds and needs. The simple act of asking implies that the provider cares about the patient as a whole person, and that goes a long way toward establishing a strong practitioner-patient relationship.

Notwithstanding what patients want, very few people actually report having been asked about religion. Only 9% of patients say they've been asked, and providers freely

---

[1] Survey respondents' responses are taken verbatim from the published study reporting the findings. See *Ann Fam Med*. 2004; 2[4]:356-361.

admit this shortcoming; only 20% of doctors report asking about religion in situations other than at the end of life.

Ideally, asking these questions would be routine in the practitioner-patient interaction. Physicians would have time to ask all the right questions, build relationships, understand each patient's expectations, and strive to meet those expectations. In that ideal world, practitioners would have the opportunity to fully know each of their patients as individuals, including their religious beliefs or lack thereof, and to use that background and knowledge when providing treatment.

But health care providers do not live in an ideal world. It is rare for a physician to have the time to acknowledge every facet of a patient's being during a routine visit — let alone during times of medical crisis.

Unfortunately, this reality doesn't align with patient expectations. It can cause frustration and dissatisfaction, affecting the doctor-patient relationship in a very real way. The challenge, therefore, is to fully understand those expectations, determine which are relevant, and then to find both time- and cost-effective ways to address them. This manual aims to help with that process.

Providers report a wide variety of barriers to addressing the spiritual concerns of patients, including[2]:

- Discomfort (e.g., "inadequate training," "discomfort with the subject matter," or "difficulty of using appropriate language");

- Time constraints (a perennial complaint);

- Misunderstanding of patients' wants ("belief that patients do not want to share spiritual concerns with physicians"); to

- Hostility ("negative attitude towards spiritual assessments").

Some practitioners simply take the position that medicine is about science and that religion has no place in it. While questions about the efficacy of spirituality and health care are open to debate, the real issue is that many patients bring religion into their treatment whether practitioners would prefer it or not. By neglecting this, health care providers can lose an important chance to provide even better care. Whatever the reason, the critical questions are not being asked and a valuable opportunity to gather vital information and build rapport with patients is being lost.

This manual is designed to help you address that situation with your own patients. As you go through it, you will find simple, time-effective ways to make religious competence part of your practice. Begin by learning about spiritual assessments and communication skills, or start exploring information about the United States' largest religious traditions.

---

[2] Physicians' responses are taken verbatim from the published study reporting the findings. See *Fam Pract.* 1999; 48:105-109.

2

Talking About Religion: Challenges and Opportunities

It's hard for many people to discuss religion, whether in their daily lives or in health care settings. Many practitioners are uncomfortable and avoid the subject with patients, colleagues, and staff.

Sometimes, this is simply because many people were raised *not* to talk about "religion and politics" in public. Other times, it is because people fear being treated poorly or differently because of their beliefs, or because they don't know the right words to use and don't want to cause offense. Whatever the reason, most people often avoid the topic, treating religion as something that not only *shouldn't* be talked about but something that there's no *need* to talk about.

In some situations—health care settings included—people *do* need to talk about it. Without these conversations, physicians and other providers risk doing themselves and their patients a disservice. Religion *is* deeply personal and, for many, it has a real impact on how they live their lives. Every day, people make decisions about what to wear, what to eat, how to interact with others, how to spend free time, and more, based on religious beliefs. Talking about religion presents real opportunities to learn important information. In health care settings, taking the time to address religion means collecting more information about patients that can help providers improve the quality of care offered. Doing this can be challenging. But the benefits, from improved outcomes to an improved bottom line, are worth it.

It does take practice to be able to have these discussions effectively and with comfort. For many people, there are real stumbling blocks to conversations about religion, including:

- Not knowing how to ask the questions;

- Being unsure of what to do with any information received;

- Worrying that the other person doesn't welcome a conversation about religion; and

- Worrying about how others will react to our beliefs.

Health care providers also have additional, unique challenges:

- Many are pressed for time, and facilities are often understaffed. It's natural for practitioners to be resistant to the idea that they *need* to add this additional, seemingly non-clinical task to already busy days.

- Most providers are not trained in why it is important to address religion. If practitioners don't see a relationship between religion and medicine, they aren't likely to expect the conversation to be valuable.

- If physicians or other providers are themselves religious, they may worry about introducing an element of coercion into the conversation that will damage the provider-patient relationships.

These challenges are real, but they're also surmountable. With education, information, effort, and a willingness to make some mistakes, practitioners can increase their comfort levels with the topic and gain a valuable tool as health care providers. This doesn't mean a physician needs to know everything there is to know about every religious tradition. There are thousands of different traditions and it's impossible to know about all of them. It *does* mean that providers should learn more about *why* these conversations are so important and how to have them respectfully.

When practitioners learn to talk about religion and use what they learn to help their patients, rewards and opportunities can result:

- The opportunity to build deeper provider-patient relationships, which often translates into greater patient loyalty and improved adherence;

- The chance to learn more about patient behaviors and how they access health care;

- The capacity to build stronger relationships among staff members; and

- The ability to break down culturally and religiously motivated barriers to health care.

Most importantly, talking with patients about religion can provide real guidance on how to treat their complaint effectively. Consider a cautionary tale that has taken place many times across the country:

> A patient enters the hospital for valve replacement surgery. Surgeons successfully replace the failing valve with a biological porcine valve. The prognosis is good and there is full expectation of a rapid recovery.

PART 1: AN INTRODUCTION TO RELIGION & HEALTH CARE

The patient's body doesn't accept the new valve. The patient is depressed and under great stress. S/he heals slowly and even starts to regress.

This outcome could have been completely different if only the providers had discussed the patient's religious beliefs and needs before proceeding with surgery: The patient was Jewish. Many observant Jews keep kosher, following dietary rules called kashruth that forbid pork. The psychological response to having a forbidden substance permanently implanted in one's body can be traumatic and, for this patient, it had a real impact on health outcomes.

This is not a one-time scenario. Many of the patients challenged with this issue had good outcomes in the end; through conversations with their providers, hospital chaplains, or their own rabbis, they were able to accept the procedures they had undergone, heal, and move on.

However, a better, healthier, less risky alternative would have been to avoid the postsurgical stress by having the conversation beforehand, perhaps involving the patient's clergyperson, or exploring other options for dealing with the underlying valve problem.

It is true. The opportunities *do* outweigh the challenges.

3

Addressing Religion in Care: Good Business Sense

Paying attention to patients' religious needs leads to stronger doctor-patient relationships and more patient-centered care—but it also makes good sense for the bottom line.

Consider what happened in Maine:
An urban hospital in an area with a substantial Muslim population noticed that Muslim women were not coming in to the hospital or its associated clinics for primary care. When they did come in, the women were reluctant patients, had poor adherence, and often failed to show up for follow-up visits. The hospital decided to do some poking around, speaking first with Muslim staff members and then reaching out to the community.

What did they discover?
Flimsy hospital gowns. Many observant Muslim women choose to dress modestly, which can range from a simple scarf tied around the head to a floor-length robe that leaves only the face or eyes visible. The observant women in this community were unwilling to access the health care facility because it meant wearing short gowns that left their neck, arms, and legs needlessly exposed.

The facility took their concerns seriously and went back to the drawing board. Continuing to work with the community, the hospital developed a gown alternative: flowing top and long, loose pants. The top and pants were loose enough to give physicians access to the patient, but provided enough coverage to satisfy the women.

The result ...
The facility noticed an immediate and lasting increase in the number of Muslim women coming in for care. Not only did the hospital's proactive approach make health care accessible for this population, but it impacted its bottom line. The patient load increased and the hospital earned a reputation in the community as a facility willing to reach out and make changes to broaden access for a marginalized population.

Such a reputation is valuable not only among the Muslim community but is also likely to influence other populations facing cultural or religious barriers to health care, further increasing the facility's market share. This hospital is now a model of best practices.

Making religio-cultural competency part of your practice has three significant bottom-line benefits as well.

As noted, it increases patient satisfaction—and loyalty. A recent study found that patients who felt their spiritual needs had been met were more likely to express satisfaction with their hospital stays *and* to return to that facility for future medical needs. In addition, patients report having greater trust in a physician who asks about religious needs. More trust translates into better adherence, which can, in turn, create a record of good medical outcomes.

There is also a strong correlation between malpractice claims and communication gaffes. Patients who feel that their providers actually listened to them and tried their best are less likely to bring malpractice claims, even when the medical outcome is poor. Religious competence and the respectful communication skills it requires is one way to build relationships that decrease lawsuits.

Second, building religious competence has a positive impact on employee relationships. Training sessions build rapport between staff members and are also a great way to identify religious tensions arising among staff. As providers increase their comfort level with different religions and gain the ability to ask questions of their patients, they also develop skills to use with colleagues, leading to a more inclusive work environment. Education in religious competence helps your staff function as an efficient team.

It also has a very direct bottom-line impact—reduced turnover. Building religious competence is an inside-out endeavor; it requires looking at how you treat patients *and* how you treat colleagues and staff. The practices of respect you show for patients become a model for the work environment.

Colleagues who feel that their whole selves are valued are more engaged, loyal colleagues. Depending on the size of your organization, turnover costs can be anywhere from 100-200% of a departing employee's salary. In the health care context, where people form relationships with their providers and a certain trust level is required, turnover creates real difficulties in continuity. This is compounded if the person leaving is a nurse, a critical position which continues to suffer a shortfall of employees.

Finally, religious competence has an additional benefit if you work in or administer a large facility: Fulfilling Joint Commission requirements. Among other things, the JCAHO standards require that you:

- Allow patients and family to express their spiritual beliefs and cultural practices, as long as there is no interference with treatment;

- Consider spiritual beliefs in patient assessment;

- Consider spiritual beliefs in managing pain; and

- Respect patients' rights to pastoral care and other spiritual services.

A strong JCAHO rating marks you as an institution that offers high-quality care. Institutionalizing religious competence is one tool you have to achieve to receive that rating.

Hopefully, your interest in religio-cultural competency comes from a desire to deepen your relationships with patients and enhance patient-centered care. But if you need more reasons to make this part of your practice, think about the business case.

4

Demographic Changes and Their Impact

Religio-cultural competence is not just something physicians and other providers need to develop to enhance their practices—it's something they need to develop because of the changing populations they are serving. A convergence of significant trends is making religio-cultural competence something health care practitioners can't afford to ignore.

IMMIGRATION TRENDS

America has always been a melting pot—a land of immigrants—and that is more true today than at any point since our founding.

Thirty years ago, just less than 5% of the population was foreign-born. That number has now more than doubled: the most recent available statistics, from the 2000 census, show that 11% of the population is foreign-born. Today, census department estimates put that number closer to 13%.

Not only are more than one-tenth of American residents foreign-born, but more people are coming to the United States from more regions of the world than ever. In 1970, the vast majority of immigrants to the United States came from Europe, with small numbers also coming from Latin America and Asia. Today, only 15% of immigrants are from Europe. The majority are from Latin America, and substantial percentages come from Asia and Africa.

In major urban areas, new Americans congregate and these numbers rise dramatically. In New York State, 20% of the population is foreign-born, while in New York City, that percentage shoots up to 29%—almost one-third of New York City's population started life outside the United States.

What do all these statistics mean for health care providers? Most obviously, it means that diverse practitioners are treating more and more diverse patient populations. Providers need a heightened sensitivity to religious and cultural differences and tools to transcend language barriers. It also means that providers' colleagues are increasingly diverse, which means learning to navigate religiously and culturally diverse workplaces; a nurse or patient aide trained outside the United States may have a different concept of what his/her job entails than one trained here.

Not only are practitioners working with more foreign patients and colleagues, but these people are coming from countries that have been underrepresented in the United States until now. When the majority of our immigrants were coming from Europe, where the majority was Christian and Jewish, assimilation into our culture (the United States is 85% Christian) was less difficult. The religious and cultural practices these immigrants brought might have been new, but would still have fit into a familiar framework.

Today, more and more immigrants are bringing minority religious traditions with which Americans may be unfamiliar. The United States now has significant Muslim, Sikh, and Buddhist populations. Increased immigration from Africa and the Caribbean brings syncretic traditions like Voudon and Candomblé. Adherents of these traditions may bring attitudes about health and illness or traditional healing methods that are foreign to US-trained providers.

AGE-RELATED TRENDS

Along with immigration, age-related trends—dealing with both the elderly and youth—are pushing religion into the limelight.

The United States is in the midst of an unprecedented aging boom. The number of residents over the age of 65, which stood at 35 million in 2000, is projected to more than double over the next 30 years. Countries around the globe are experiencing a similar phenomenon.

As Americans age, it may become more important for their health care providers to address this critical component of patients' personal identity. Providers will be seeing older patients more frequently. Some will have long-term or degenerative illnesses; others may need to enter long-term care facilities. They and their families will face difficult end-of-life decisions.

As people age, their relationships to religion shift. Some people fall away from their faith, but many more turn toward it as a source of strength and comfort as illness sets in and friends and loved ones begin to pass away. Sixty-two percent of Americans say that religion is very important in their lives, but among people 65 and older, that percentage jumps up to 73%. Thus, providers will not only be spending more time treating the elderly, but will be spending more time with patients to whom religion is a significant source of strength (and, potentially, health).

Young Americans are also becoming more outspoken about religion. An ongoing study of U.S. college students shows that a full 83% are affiliated with some religious denomination, and 70% say that religion is an important part of their lives. Forty percent say it is important to follow religious teachings in their everyday lives.

These young religious people are not only becoming our patients, but also our colleagues.

RELIGIOSITY

Among Western nations, the United States is one of the most deeply religious, if not *the* most deeply religious. Studies consistently show that around 90% of Americans believe in a God, and 75% of us characterize our outlook on life as "somewhat religious" or "very religious." Only 16% report having a "largely secular" outlook, meaning that religion is not a major factor in their day-to-day lives.

Religious beliefs are not always private and personal, either. Almost one-half of Americans report talking to co-workers about religion at least weekly and more than one-half say that religion has a role in interactions with colleagues and the decisions made at work. More significantly for health care providers, 41% of Americans report that religious beliefs have directly influenced a health care decision they've made for themselves or a loved one.

As all these trends continue, America's diversity—religious, cultural, and otherwise—will continue to increase. Being a competent provider in this multicultural world increasingly requires that practitioners understand how to navigate the diverse beliefs and practices of their patient populations.

5
····

Not Just Religion: Spirituality and Patient Care

While some researchers are assessing the power of religious beliefs and/or spirituality to impact healing, this manual does not address those questions. As such, our goal is neither to promote nor to denigrate the power of religion and spirituality, but rather to emphasize how they can affect patient decision making and how this may require practitioners to reconsider how they respond in order to ensure the best health outcomes. Thus, this manual affirmatively takes the position that practitioners should not promote or impose religion or spirituality on a patient, but rather that they should be alert when it is playing a role in the patient's health care and respond appropriately.

Given the foregoing, much of this manual deals with what are commonly called "organized religions" and how practicing those religions can affect health care decisions. Our focus has not been on what is commonly defined as spirituality. Nonetheless, it is important to acknowledge that spirituality, both within and outside of organized religion and its beliefs, is also important in the lives of many people. How individuals manifest spirituality is as individual as how they might manifest their religion; both spiritual and religious practices can influence decisions and compliance with medical treatment. It is as important for providers to recognize this component of personal identity and how it can affect patient care as it is to understand the laws of kashruth or halal.

DEFINING OUR TERMS: RELIGION AND SPIRITUALITY

Although the words "religion" and "spirituality" are often used interchangeably, they actually refer to two different concepts. Most of this manual focuses on organized religions, that is, belief systems with agreed upon components: sacred texts, doctrines, deities, and practices.

All religions may not include every one of those components, but they have at least some element or tradition that is widely shared among fellow believers in the particular religious community or denomination. For example, Shintō has no holy books, but has agreed upon beliefs, rituals, and holidays. Native American religions differ widely from tribe to tribe, but each has a world-view and concept of humanity's relationship to nature. Islam, Judaism, Christianity, and Sikhism have sacred texts, shared beliefs, and shared rituals.

In contrast, "spirituality" typically refers to one's *personal* relationship to a higher power, to others, or to the world. As opposed to the tenets of organized religions, which exist independently of any individual believer, spirituality is even more highly individualized. Because it is so self-directed and is not bound by any agreed upon religious principles, it is also flexible: A person can be both religious *and* spiritual (e.g., a committed Christian who attends church follows the tenets of Christianity and also meditates individually to deepen his/her relationship to God), or spiritual but not religious (e.g., someone who believes in some higher power but does not subscribe to any particular religion's view concerning that power). Personal spirituality may be a completely internal experience, or may influence a person's actions and behavior. It can also be totally secular. A person may not believe in any kind of divine higher power, but may find comfort, support, and meaning in a range of practices including meditation, music, or running.

WHAT DOES SPIRITUALITY LOOK LIKE?

Because it is so highly individual, spirituality can look like anything at all—or nothing. Personal spirituality may involve prayer, meditation, or yoga. It can include specific rituals or behaviors that have roots in a religious tradition or that are unique to the person. There may be outward manifestations, like keeping a vegetarian diet, or no discernible signs at all.

WHAT DOES THIS MEAN FOR PROVIDERS?

Although varieties of personal spirituality are vast, understanding patients' needs comes down to the same respectful communication needed when discussing more overtly religious topics.

In theory, discussing spirituality is no different from discussing religion. After all, all adherents of a particular religion don't believe and practice in exactly the same way — no two Hindus or Sikhs practice their faiths identically—and good communication is required to understand each person's particular needs. Thus, practitioners need to talk to their patients to understand whether and to what extent spirituality has meaning for them, their sources of strength, how they cope, and whether there are particular practices or observations that are important to them that might impact their health care behaviors or decision making.

The spiritual assessment tools suggested in this manual are deliberately broad so that they apply to discussions of religion and/or personal spirituality. Here are a few of the questions that will be more important when discussing personal spirituality:

- What gives your life meaning?

- What are your sources of hope?

- Do you have any beliefs or practices that help you cope with stress?

- Does faith or belief have any importance in your life?

- Are there any spiritual practices you have that I, as your health care provider, should know about?

Reading through some spiritual assessment tools will give you more ideas for ways to have these conversations.

ONE TOOL: THE RELAXATION RESPONSE

Among the groundbreaking work in this area is the research of Dr. Herbert Benson of Harvard Medical School, who uses a tool called the Relaxation Response to reduce stress (which is increasingly being associated with any number of medical conditions and is known to exacerbate illness and delay healing). Although the Relaxation Response is useful for any patient, religious, spiritual, or atheist/agnostic, we discuss it here because it may be of particular use for non-religious or spiritually inclined patients who do not have a religious community, rituals, or prayer upon which they rely for comfort or stress relief.

The relaxation response is a "physical state of deep rest that changes the physical and emotional responses to stress... and the opposite of the fight or flight response."[3] Studied and outlined by Dr. Herbert Benson of Harvard Medical School, one of the pioneers in researching the mind-body relationship, the Relaxation Response is a calm, stress-free state brought about by a simple meditation on a word or phrase. Dr. Benson has established that a reduction of stress can improve healing, bringing about better health outcomes.

According to Benson, the key elements needed to invoke the Relaxation Response are:

A Quiet Environment
Ideally, the patient should be in a quiet, calm environment with as few distractions as possible; this may not always be possible for hospitalized or bedridden patients. A calm setting also makes it easier to eliminate distracting thoughts. For a religious or spiritual person, this might be a religious setting.

---

[3] Benson H. *The Relaxation Response.* New York: HarperTorch; 1976, p. 4.

A Mental Device

A constant, repetitive stimulus — a sound, word, or phrase repeated silently or aloud — is used to focus the mind and helps to remove the patient from focusing on everyday thoughts. One of the major challenges for eliciting the Response is that the mind wanders, and repetition of a word or phrase helps break through those distracting thoughts. Attention to the rhythm of breathing is also useful.

A religious person may choose a word related to his/her faith. A non-religious but spiritual person or an atheist or agnostic may select a word that has personal meaning or a random word used only for meditation purposes.

A Passive Attitude

This is the most important element needed to create the Relaxation Response. When distracting thoughts occur, the patient is instructed not to dwell on them, returning instead to the repetition of the mental device.

A Comfortable Position

A comfortable posture is needed to avoid distracting muscle tension. Patients can try sitting, lying down, or the yoga "lotus" position. In any case, the patient should feel comfortable and relaxed.

THE BOTTOM LINE

Patients bring an endless variety of religious and spiritual practices with them when they visit the doctor or enter a hospital or long-term care facility, and not all of them stem from a recognized, organized religion. To offer optimal, patient-centered care, practitioners must ask the right questions and learn what patients are turning to for meaning or as a guide to their health care decisions.

PART II

• • • •

How to Understand Your Patients

• • • •

Spiritual Assessment Instruments

Understanding Your Patients: Communication Skills

When Religion Becomes Relevant: Spiritual Journeys

Incorporating Spiritual Assessments into Treatment Plans

Checklists and Organizational Tools

PART 2: HOW TO UNDERSTAND YOUR PATIENTS

1
. . . .
Spiritual Assessment Instruments

There are a number of different patient assessment tools designed to help providers learn more about patients' religious and cultural beliefs and how they may impact health care. Some are relatively direct, asking pointed questions about religion and spirituality, while others are broader and encourage the patient to open up and discuss his/her religious understanding of illness.

Each of these approaches may be useful, depending on the circumstances and the patient. For example, providers may want to ask different types of questions of a patient who is being admitted to the hospital for potentially life-threatening surgery than to one who is coming to a group practice for a routine check-up.

We provide these tools here as a resource for you to use or as the basis for creating your own model.

PART 2: HOW TO UNDERSTAND YOUR PATIENTS

FICA: A Spiritual Self-Assessment Tool[4]

The acronym FICA can help structure questions in taking a personal spiritual history. Broad questions help the provider draw out information about significant religious or personal beliefs that may affect health and health care, family and community structure, and other information that helps providers build strong provider-patient relationships:

F   **FAITH AND BELIEF**
"Do you consider yourself spiritual or religious?" or "Do you have spiritual beliefs that help you cope with stress?" If the patient responds, "No," the physician might ask, "What gives your life meaning?" For some patients for whom religion does not play an important role, the answer might be family, career, or nature.

I   **IMPORTANCE**
"What importance does your faith or belief have in your life? Have your beliefs influenced how you take care of yourself in this illness? What role do your beliefs play in regaining your health?"

C   **COMMUNITY**
"Are you part of a spiritual or religious community? Is this of support to you, and how? Is there a group of people you really love or who are important to you?" Communities such as churches, temples, and mosques, or a group of like-minded friends can serve as strong support systems for some patients.

A   **ADDRESS IN CARE**
"How would you like me, your health care provider, to address these issues in your care?"

---

[4] Created by the George Washington Institute for Spirituality and Health at The George Washington University.

HOPE Questions for a Formal Spiritual Assessment in a Medical Interview[5]

The HOPE questions were developed as a teaching tool to help medical students, residents, and practicing physicians begin the process of incorporating a spiritual assessment into the medical interview. They cover the basic areas of inquiry for physicians to use in formal spiritual assessments.

H — **HOPE**
What are the patient's basic spiritual resources and sources of hope? These may be religion or, as in the previous tool, something else.

O — **ORGANIZED RELIGION**
Is organized religion an important part of the patient's life? Is there a religious community to which the patient is attached?

P — **PERSONAL SPIRITUALITY AND PRACTICES**
"Do you have personal spiritual beliefs? What aspects of your personal spirituality or spiritual practice are more helpful to you in times of stress?"

E — **EFFECT ON MEDICAL CARE AND END-OF-LIFE**
"Are there any specific practices I should know about, as your provider? How has your current situation affected your spirituality or religious life?"

---

[5] Developed by Dr. Harold Koenig of the Center for Spirituality, Theology and Health at Duke University; printed in *Am Fam Phys.* 2001; 63:81-89.

Kleinman's Questions for Culturally Sensitive Interviewing[6]

The Kleinman questions are designed to help the provider elicit the patient's perspective on the causes of his/her illness. Instead of focusing directly on religious or cultural needs, they explore the patient's understanding of his/her problem, how it is impacting his/her daily life, and what types of treatment the patient wants. Indirectly, the provider learns a great deal about the patient's religious beliefs and needs, uncovers potential barriers to treatment, and learns about alternative remedies the patient may seek.

1. "What do you think caused your problem?"

2. "Why do you think it started when it did?"

3. "What do you think your sickness does to you?"

4. "How severe is your sickness? Do you think it will last a long time or will it be better soon, in your opinion?"

5. "What are the chief problems your sickness has caused for you?"

6. "What do you fear most about your sickness?"

7. "What kind of treatment would you like to have?"

8. "What are the most important results you hope to get from treatment?"

---

[6] Kleinman A, Eisenberg L, Good B. Culture, illness, and health care: Clinical lessons from anthropologic and cross-cultural research. *Ann Int Med*, 1978; 88[2]: 251-258.

The ETHNIC Model[7]

Like the Kleinman questions, the ETHNIC model helps the provider explore the patient's religious and cultural understanding of illness:

E   **EXPLANATION**
"What do you think may be the reason you have these symptoms? What do friends, family, or others say about these symptoms? Do you know anyone else who has had or who has this kind of problem? Have you heard about/read/seen it on TV/radio/newspaper?" (If patient cannot offer explanation, ask him/her what most concerns him/her about the problem.)

T   **TREATMENT**
"What kinds of medicines, home remedies, or other treatments have you tried for this illness? Is there anything you eat, drink, or do (or avoid) on a regular basis to stay healthy? Tell me about it. What kind of treatment are you seeking from me?"

H   **HEALERS**
"Have you sought any advice from alternative/traditional or folk healers, friends, or other people (non-doctors) for help with your problems? Tell me about it."

N   **NEGOTIATE**
Negotiate options that will be mutually acceptable to you and your patient and that do not contradict, but rather incorporate your patient's beliefs.

I   **INTERVENTION**
Determine an intervention with your patient. This may include incorporation of alternative treatments, spirituality, and healers, as well as other cultural practices (e.g., foods eaten or avoided both in general and when sick).

C   **COLLABORATION**
Collaborate with the patient, family members, other health care team members, healers, and community resources.

---

[7] Levin SJ, Like RC, Gottlieb JE. Useful clinical interviewing mnemonics. *Patient Care*. 2000;34: 189-190.

2

Understanding Your Patients: Communication Skills

How questions are asked is just as important as what questions are asked. Insensitive use of a spiritual assessment can irritate, annoy, or offend a patient. Before beginning a patient interview, keep these guidelines in mind:

Recognize your own lens

Before starting to talk with others about their religious beliefs and needs, it's critical to be aware of one's own religious and cultural lens—this lens influences the way we hear and understand others. Are you highly religious, or do you yourself pray when you're ill? Do you have any opinions about other religions or people who do not follow a particular religious belief or practice? Do you believe that the practice of medicine is a strictly scientific endeavor and that religion plays no role?

Two identically trained and competent physicians holding different beliefs will hear two very different things when talking with the same patient about his/her religious and cultural needs.

Doctors and nurses certainly have personal characteristics other than as "health care providers," and are not expected to be completely neutral service providers, but providers should be aware of any beliefs they hold that might impact the way they hear patients' concerns.

Take responsibility

Chaplains are not the only people in a hospital who need to care about patients' religious needs. While religious patients may well want to see a chaplain or clergyperson, that's not the full extent of incorporating religion into a treatment plan. Does the patient have special dietary needs? Does s/he have religious objections to any medications or procedures? Often, a patient's beliefs and practices have a direct impact on care.

Don't assume anything in your questions

Always ask inclusive, open-ended questions. The goal of these questions is always to start a conversation with the patient from which we can learn—not to cut him/her off with a question to which s/he can't respond.

For example, ask, "Do you have spiritual beliefs or practices that are important to you?" or "Do you have religious beliefs?"

Don't ask, "What spiritual practices are important to you?" or "What is your religion?". The question, "What is your religion?" can be highly alienating to a patient who is an atheist or agnostic, or one who follows his/her own form of personal spirituality.

Don't assume anything in your patient's answers

Knowing that your patient is Buddhist or Hindu doesn't actually tell you very much about that particular patient. People practice their faiths in an infinite variety of ways, and a provider can never assume that a Buddhist patient will reject narcotics or that a Hindu patient is a vegetarian. Use such broad answers as a starting point to learn more about how that individual observes his/her religion and what his/her needs are.

Embrace the opportunity to learn

Knowing that a patient is Muslim is only helpful if you know something about Islamic beliefs and practices and then how the particular individual applies them. Don't be afraid to ask clarifying questions or seek more in-depth explanations.

No one speaks for everyone

What you learn from one patient about his/her religious or spiritual practice *may or may not* apply to your next encounter with a person from the same religion. Remember, religious or spiritual identities have a vast spectrum of difference in belief and practice.

Notice other indicators: context clues and body language

Not all patients welcome discussions of spirituality with their health care providers. Pay close attention to the patient's comfort level, and don't press a disinterested or hostile patient.

Context clues are equally important; a patient may not know which of his/her practices a health care provider would want to know about, and may unknowingly withhold information. Are there certain foods s/he refuses to eat? Is s/he more comfortable with female providers? Behavioral clues can help indicate what to ask to fill in the gaps.

Re-assess periodically

A patient's spiritual needs sometimes change as s/he enters different stages of illness or different stages of life in general. A healthy incoming patient may not want visits from clergy, but a deteriorating patient may welcome such a visit, and vice versa. If you have long-term relationships with patients, or have a patient who is hospitalized for a period of time, re-assess periodically to make sure you're not missing anything.

"No" is a valid answer

Many patients do not identify with any spiritual or religious belief or practice, or choose not to bring this dimension of their identity into the health care setting. Showing respect for this answer is critical. "No" is not an indication that the patient would not welcome accommodation or support in another form.

Be curious
Although the patient may be the most obvious source of information about the patient's own religious tradition, part of the onus for learning more is also on you. It is inappropriate to expect your patient to educate you on every facet of his/her religion. Take responsibility to improve the care you offer by seeking out information on a patient's religious tradition—you can use this manual as a starting place.

Don't check it and forget it
A spiritual assessment is not just a checklist, but a way to build a relationship and create a comfort level with a patient while gathering useful information. Don't be afraid to go into more depth or ask for additional information if a particular topic seems to be important to your patient.

3

When Religion Becomes Relevant: Spiritual Journeys

A healthy 18-year-old patient visiting a physician for a routine checkup may not want to discuss—or even care about—religion. That same patient, now a 65-year-old Buddhist with a dedicated meditation practice and Parkinson's disease, may very well want to discuss his religious aversion to taking a medication that alters his brain chemistry when he meets with a physician. To provide religiously competent care, it is important to pay attention to the life stages in which patients find themselves and to reflect on whether it provides any information that might be pertinent to a patient's religious needs and his/her health care.

As people progress through the different stages of their lives, their relationship to religion often changes. This can mean that at different life stages, a person may consider himself or herself an intimate part of a practicing religious community and at other times an individual devoted to his/her own spirituality. Self-perception and community affiliations can change as attitudes toward religion change. As a health care provider, these can be additional indicators about how religion functions in a patient's life and its impact on his/her health care.

Many theorists have articulated theories of different life stages, each with their own life tasks and issues, and each with their own positive and negative aspects (for some examples of different theories see the resources). What is key (regardless of which theory is used) is that the practitioner needs to appreciate how different events in a patient's life cycle can implicate religion, so that the provider can shift the way s/he relates to and treats that patient.

One way a patient's relationship to religion evolves is through the maturation and aging process. As people age and develop the critical thinking skills to make their own decisions about how to relate to the world, their relationship with religion and reliance on religious dictates may change. A young girl who attends church regularly with her parents at age 5 might continue going, stop going, or become even more devout at age 15, when she is able to evaluate her position for herself. Things may shift again when she goes to college, moves out of the house, partners with a spouse, or decides to have children.

For the provider who has an ongoing relationship with a patient, being aware of these shifts can have a real impact on both rapport and treatment. An 18-year-old observant Jehovah's Witness might not want a surgical procedure requiring a blood transfusion. That same patient might go away to college and become a Taoist, and be perfectly willing to accept the procedure the next time s/he visits. A few years later, s/he may return to the community and again take up his/her childhood beliefs. A provider needs to be able to recognize these shifts to ensure that the care offered is consistent with the patient's evolving religious needs and practices.

Religious shifts can also happen in tandem with major life events like moving, going away to college, marriage, childbirth, divorce, illness, and death. Turbulent life events might cause a patient to adopt or adhere more tightly to religious beliefs, or to turn away from a faith tradition s/he perceives as useless. A patient for whom religion is not usually very important may suddenly turn to it when admitted to the hospital for major surgery. Again, a provider will need to be attuned to these shifts and understand how they will impact the way that patient accesses health care.

These changes in one's relation to religion can be characterized as a person's spiritual journey. For a practitioner to be religiously competent, it is necessary to recognize not only that adherents of a particular faith may believe and practice differently from their co-congregationalists, but also that there will also be great variation among practitioners at different stages in their lives.

To make the idea of spiritual journeys more concrete, it may be helpful to reflect on one's own journey. How has your own life journey had an impact on your religious journey? Have you yourself become more or less attached to religion over the course of your life? What was going on in your life at the time that may have influenced this shift? What connections can you draw from your personal experience to help inform you about others?

Below are some questions to help you learn more about your patient's current life stage and how it may (or may not) affect the care you provide. Keep this list with your patient intake and history materials, and refer to it when appropriate.

- What is the patient's current religious affiliation? What are the implications of the patient's religious beliefs for the treatment you recommend, if any?

- Has the patient's religious affiliation changed over the course of his/her life? Since his/her last visit with you? Does this suggest any additional religious factors to take into account?

PART 2: HOW TO UNDERSTAND YOUR PATIENTS

- ❧ If the patient is married or partnered, is the patient's spouse/partner of the same religious tradition? How does the couple navigate this? Is the patient's spouse/partner equipped to help the patient meet his/her religious needs?

- ❧ Is the patient facing a major change in health status (e.g., diagnosis with a long-term condition)?

- ❧ Has the patient recently dealt with a major life change, such as:

    - Going away to college or leaving home;

    - Changing jobs;

    - Losing a job;

    - Moving;

    - Getting married;

    - Getting divorced;

    - Becoming pregnant;

    - Giving birth; or

    - Sending a child to college or having a child leave home (in other words, become an empty nester)?

    - Has the patient recently dealt with the major illness or death of a loved one?

SPIRITUAL JOURNEYS: RESOURCES

• • • •

Erikson, Erik H. *The Life Cycle Completed.* W.W. Norton & Company, 1998.
An overview of the nine life stages identified by Erikson, one of the fathers of modern psychology.

Thomas, L. Eugene & Eisenhandler, Susan A., eds. *Aging and the Religious Dimension.* Auburn House, 1994.
Original theory and research exploring the role religion plays in the lives of the elderly.

Gilligan, Carol. *In a Different Voice.* Harvard University Press, 1993.
Feminist exploration of the differences in moral development between boys/men and girls/women.

Opper, Sylvia, & Ginsburg, Herbert P. *Piaget's Theory of Intellectual Development.* Prentice Hall, 1987.
A concise introduction to Jean Piaget's groundbreaking theory of stages of cognitive development from infancy to adulthood.

4

Incorporating Spiritual Assessments into Treatment Plans

Understanding the importance of religious competence and asking the right questions of patients are great first steps—but they are just that, first steps. Valuable information is only valuable when it is used properly. In this case, the information you collect on a patient's religious beliefs and practices becomes useful when it is incorporated into the treatment plan in a real way.

An intake form may state that a patient is Jewish and keeps kosher. Unless that is clearly communicated to the nutritionist responsible for the meal plans, the nurses' aide who assists with dressing and bathing, the pharmacist who would otherwise use a non-kosher gelatin-based capsule to deliver medicine, or the surgeon preparing to install a porcine valve in the patient, the information is not doing the patient any good. But ignoring it could do harm.

Each patient and medical issue is different. A one-size-fits-all approach to integrating a patient's religious needs into his/her treatment plan will fall short, and this manual cannot provide an exact road map for any particular patient. Instead, this tool can help practitioners explore the many categories in which religion and health care interface and prompt you to think about tailoring the care provided to offer a more whole-person, patient-centered experience.

Some of these categories will be obvious—hospitals routinely inquire into patients' dietary needs and many are able to provide certified kosher or halal meals. Some categories are less apparent—many providers may not see informed consent as anything other than a patient issue, even though the patient may want the decision to be made by or at least to first receive the approval of a parent, spouse, elder, or religious leader before consenting to a procedure.

The assessment tools below are designed to help you keep track of the obvious and the not-so-obvious issues. Print a copy of the one-pager to keep in your office, at a nurses' station, or in any other appropriate location in your facility as a quick reference. Keep copies of the checklist with your other intake and patient assessment materials. With each new patient or admission, run through the checklist to identify areas in which attention to religious belief or practice may be important. As the various providers with whom the patient interacts learn more about the patient, add information to the document. Keep the completed checklist in the patient's file, and make sure all appropriate providers are alerted to potential issues.

5

Checklists and Organizational Tools

RELIGION & PATIENT CARE: INTERSECTIONS

Struggling with a patient and not sure how to proceed? *Maybe there's a religious issue in play.* Religion isn't just about private spiritual beliefs—it can involve beliefs and practices that impact how a patient accesses health care.

Here are the many areas in which religion can intersect with health care. Is there an area in which your patient might have an unaddressed religious need? Keep a copy of this checklist posted in an accessible place, and consult it when appropriate.

- Dietary Requirements
- Dress & Modesty
- Gender & Modesty
- Hygiene & Washing Requirements
- Informed Consent & Patient Decision Making
- Prayer & Ritual Observances
- Traditional & Alternative Remedies
- Reproductive Health & Family Planning
- Pregnancy & Birth
- Blood & Blood Products
- Organ Transplants & Donations
- Acceptance of Drugs & Certain Procedures
- End of Life

PART 2: HOW TO UNDERSTAND YOUR PATIENTS

RELIGION & PATIENT CARE: INTERSECTIONS
Keep copies of this checklist with other patient assessment materials.

Dietary Requirements
- Does the patient keep kosher or halal, or have other religiously motivated food restrictions? If so, are there medically necessary restricted foods, or medicines derived from restricted foods? How has this been explained to the patient? Is there a medically sound alternative?

- Is the patient observing a religious fast? Is the patient refusing solids, liquids, or both? Is a fast interfering with treatment or worsening the patient's health?

- Is the patient consuming any particular traditional cultural or religious foods? Is the patient medically cleared to consume these foods?

Dress & Modesty

- Does the patient wear religious garb? If this garb is not appropriate for a health care setting, are there alternatives that meet religious modesty requirements?

- Does the patient wear religious symbols? If the symbols must be removed for treatment, are they removed with care?

- Do providers and staff understand how to handle and store any religious garb or symbols that must be removed?

Gender & Modesty

- Does the patient prefer to be examined by practitioners of the same sex? If one is not available, would the patient like a relative or chaperone present?

- Are there particular topics that a patient will not discuss with a provider of the opposite sex or that a patient will be reluctant to discuss at all (e.g., sexual activity)?

Hygiene & Washing Requirements
- Does the patient have any religious beliefs around washing or bathing? Is there a reason why it may not be recommended for the patient to bathe or shower, and has this been explained?

- Does the patient wash any parts of his/her body before or after particular events, like prayers, mealtimes, or trips to the bathroom? Does the patient need assistance with this? Is staff prepared to assist patients with limited mobility?

- Does the patient have religious beliefs concerning growing or maintaining hair? Does the patient require periodic brushing or washing of the hair? Is staff prepared to assist patients with limited mobility?

Informed Consent & Patient Decision Making

- Is there anyone other than the patient who should be consulted when major medical decisions are being made? Although the decision is ultimately the patient's, might bringing in a spouse or parent, elder, or religious leader to approve of treatment improve patient adherence and compliance?

Prayer & Ritual Observances

- Are there any holy days within the patient's tradition that will fall during his/her hospital stay? Does the facility provide assistance in observing this tradition (e.g., by holding a worship service, providing a special meal, etc)? If not, might the patient want to be connected to his/her clergy person, a religious leader of his/her denomination, or a chaplain?

- Has the patient brought any ritual objects with him/her? Does staff understand how to handle these objects if necessary? If any of the objects are problematic (e.g., candles or incense), have alternatives been explored?

- Is there support for patients with limited mobility who wish to attend a worship service, pray, or otherwise engage in a religious ceremony or ritual with which they will need assistance?

Traditional & Alternative Remedies

- Is the patient using any traditional or alternative remedies (e.g., herbal medicines) in conjunction with standard medical treatment? What remedies and for how long? Might this alternative remedy be contraindicated, given the patient's prognosis or treatment plan? Has this been explained to the patient and his/her family?

- Would the patient prefer to have alternative or traditional remedies incorporated into his/her treatment? Would the patient's compliance be improved if alternative or traditional remedies are incorporated into his/her treatment? Is staff prepared to work with traditional healers?

Reproductive Health & Family Planning

- Is the patient prepared to discuss reproductive and sexual health issues openly? What would help the patient to be more comfortable? Does the patient's religious or cultural background mandate that s/he have a chaperone or see a same-sex provider?

- Does the patient have religious views on contraception, abortion, or any other relevant procedure (e.g., in vitro fertilization, sterilization)? How will these affect treatment or other recommendations?

Pregnancy & Birth

- Does the patient have any religion-specific practices or beliefs associated with pregnancy, such as particular foods that should be eaten or rituals to perform? Is there anything in these practices that might be contraindicated?

- Does the patient have any religion-specific practices associated with labor and birth, such as particular foods that should be eaten, rituals to perform, people to assist, traditional remedies for a problematic labor? Are any of these contraindicated? If not, can they be incorporated?

- Are there any religious rituals that must be performed upon or shortly after birth? Is staff aware of this, and are they prepared to facilitate them (e.g., by providing space or materials)?

Blood & Blood Products
- Does the patient have religious beliefs that restrict the use of blood or blood products? If blood or blood products would usually be necessary for a particular treatment or procedure, have the alternatives been explored?

Organ Transplants & Donations

- Does the patient or his/her family have any religious beliefs that influence their willingness to accept a donor organ or agree to donate an organ?

- Are there any rituals that occur when an organ is donated or accepted? Is staff aware of them, and are they prepared to facilitate them (e.g., by providing space or materials)?

Acceptance of Drugs & Certain Procedures
- Does the patient have a religious objection to a particular drug, for example, against drugs that contain alcohol, narcotics, or another forbidden substance?

- Is there a religious reason for objecting to a particular treatment, for example, against non-essential procedures occurring on a holy day?

- Have staff explored alternatives with patients?

End of Life

- Are there traditional religious rituals performed for patients nearing death? Is staff aware of them, and are they prepared to facilitate them (e.g., by providing space or materials)?

- Is staff aware of any religious requirements governing how a body is handled after death? In particular, has staff inquired whether the body should be washed?

- If any religiously motivated end-of-life requirements are problematic (e.g., because they are against the law or hospital policy), have the issues been clearly explained to family, friends, and other visitors? Might a religious leader or chaplain be brought in to help discuss alternatives?

PART III

••••

**Religions of the World &
Their Applications to Health Care**

••••

Judaism

Christianity

Islam

Buddhism

Hinduism

Sikhism

Shintō

Traditional Chinese

American Indian/Alaska Native

Afro-Caribbean

PART 3: RELIGIONS OF THE WORLD & THEIR APPLICATIONS TO HEALTH CARE

1. Judaism

Overview FAQ

1. When, where, and how did Judaism originate?

Jewish tradition teaches that the religion began circa 2000 BCE, with a *covenant* (divine agreement) between G-d [8] and Abraham, the patriarch and progenitor of Jews. The Jewish people originated in the vicinity of what is now referred to as the Middle East, specifically Israel and Egypt.

According to Jewish tradition, Abraham was the first person to recognize and worship the one true G-d. In return, G-d promised him many offspring, who today are the Jewish people. According to the Hebrew Bible, the Jews were united by Moses, a prophet who brought them out of slavery in Egypt, led them back to Israel, and gave them laws that he received from G-d.

2. Does Judaism have sacred texts? What are they called?

Jewish tradition teaches that the *Torah* is the preeminent source of Jewish law and tradition. The word Torah, or "instruction," refers to the first five books of the Hebrew Bible. The entire Bible is called *Tanakh*. It tells the story of humanity from the creation of the earth until the Jewish people are united under Moses; it also contains ethical precepts, stories, and collections of law. It is considered to be the word of G-d as revealed to Moses.

The Tanakh contains the Torah, along with two other collections, the *Nevi'im* (or "prophets") and the *kethuvim* (or "writings"). The Nevi'im covers Jewish history post-Moses, while the kethuvim includes history, guidance, and poetry.

The *Talmud* is equally important. It is a written record of oral laws and rabbinic discussions that were first compiled circa 200 CE–500 CE. The Talmud, which comments on and interprets the Hebrew Bible, deals mainly with Jewish law, ethics, customs, and history.

3. What are the core beliefs of Judaism?

Judaism is based on the principles and ethics embodied in the Tanakh and the Talmud. Although there are a variety of belief systems within Judaism, there are common

---

[8] It is forbidden for a Jew to write the name of God in such a way that destruction of the paper (or other medium) will destroy the word. For this reason, G-d is often used as an alternative. Although not all Jews follow this proscription, this chapter renders the word as "G-d" out of respect for that practice.

principles that are widely accepted. Central to the Jewish faith is the belief that there is a single, unique G-d who is incorporeal, eternal, and exclusively worthy of being worshipped. Traditional Jews believe that G-d created the heavens and earth and all their inhabitants, and continues to oversee them.

Judaism also teaches that Abraham's covenant resulted in a personal relationship between G-d and the Jewish people. Consequently, Jews often share a sense of community and responsibility with and for one another.

Additionally, Orthodox and Conservative Jews believe in a Messianic age of peace and justice (heralded by the Jewish Messiah) that will eventually arrive, uniting all of creation in brotherhood and resurrecting the dead.

4. What are the core practices of Judaism?

There are laws set forth in the Jewish scriptures that believers may choose to follow for nearly every aspect of daily life, including mourning rituals, dress, diet, business ethics, marriage, and more. The goal of observing these practices is to embody the values of the faith in one's relationship with G-d and other people. The strictness of observance and the emphasis on certain practices vary among the different branches of Judaism.

The Jewish Sabbath (*Shabbat*) is the most holy day in Judaism, and commemorates both G-d's day of rest after creating the world and G-d freeing the Jewish people from slavery in Egypt. Shabbat officially begins just before sunset on Fridays. It is a day of rest, renewal, and family enjoyment. Highly observant Jews do not work, drive a car, operate an elevator, speak on the phone, turn on a light, operate a stove, etc on Shabbat. But almost all Jews view Shabbat as a special day.

5. What are Judaism's important holidays? How are they celebrated?

Holidays occur in accordance with the Jewish calendar, a lunar calendar. Most commemorate interactions between G-d and the Jewish people. Since Jews were an agricultural people, some holidays are agricultural in origin, celebrating harvests, planting, and the season of rain; eventually, they acquired more spiritual meanings. Two significant holidays called the High Holy Days, *Rosh Hashanah* and *Yom Kippur*, occur in the fall.

- **Rosh Hashanah** is the Jewish New Year and commemorates the creation of the world. It is the beginning of a 10-day period of penitence and spiritual renewal and is celebrated with prayers and religious services.

- **Yom Kippur**, the "Day of Atonement," is the most solemn day of the Jewish calendar. Most or all of the day is spent fasting, and in worship and contemplation, seeking forgiveness of one's sins against G-d and one's fellow humans. Repentance, charity, and acts of loving-kindness are stressed.

- **Passover** is perhaps the most beloved holiday. It is an eight-day festival marking Moses' liberation of the Israelites from slavery in Egypt, and begins with a ritual dinner (*seder*) with foods symbolizing slavery and freedom, story-telling, songs, and celebration.

Other important holidays include *Purim*, (the story of Queen Esther); *Shavuot* (commemorating the giving of the Ten Commandments); *Sukkot* (commemorating the years of wandering in the desert); and *Hanukkah* (commemorating the victory of the Maccabees for freedom of religion, the re-dedication of the Temple in Jerusalem, and the miracle of the oil). One recently inaugurated holiday recalls significant events in contemporary Jewish history: *Yom Ha-Shoah* commemorates the destruction of Jewish life during the Holocaust of World War II.

5. How many Jews are there in the United States? Are they located in a particular region?

Approximately 5–6 million people in the United States self-identify as Jewish. The largest Jewish populations are in the Boston-New York Corridor, Florida, and California.

6. What are the main sects or denominations within Judaism?

The three commonly recognized schools of Judaism are Orthodox, Reform, and Conservative Judaism. The American Jewish population includes a substantial number of *Hasidic* Jews.

- **Orthodox Judaism** teaches that all 613 laws in the Torah and the Talmud are binding, including strict observance of the Sabbath, fasting on specified occasions, modest dress and head coverings, and a diet that is in accordance with Jewish law. Additionally, Orthodox Jews may pray throughout the day for acts as varied as eating a meal, wearing new clothes, washing hands, or lighting candles.

- **Hasidism** is a small but noteworthy Orthodox movement. Its hallmark is meticulous adherence to the laws, intensive Torah study, and joyful singing and celebration. Many Hasidic Jews prefer separation from all non-Jewish society. One of the largest branches of Hasidism in the United States is the Lubavitch. Lubavitchers are known for setting up Jewish community centers (usually called *Chabad Houses*) that provide educational and outreach activities for the observant and for the non-observant.

- **Conservative** Judaism teaches that the laws from G-d set forth in the Torah are binding but evolve over time. A central Council of Rabbis debates major ethical and legal issues, and Conservative Jews are expected to follow their informed decisions.

- **Reform** Judaism teaches that the laws in the Torah are guidelines that need to be adapted to historical, cultural, and societal change. There is latitude among believers as to which guidelines they will follow in their own lives. There is a strong emphasis on social action for justice and tikkun olam, "healing the world."

- Smaller, but influential movements within Judaism include **Reconstructionism**, based on the concept that Judaism is more an emerging religious civilization than a group of beliefs, and the Jewish Renewal Movement, a "post-denominational" movement stressing study and creative ritual.

• • • •

Intersections with Health Care: FAQ

1. Does Judaism have a particular view about what causes illness? Are there illness-related rituals?

Judaism strikes a balance between recognizing purely medical explanations for illness and viewing it as part of a divine plan. The Talmud, one of the main sources of Jewish law, emphasizes the sanctity of human life; it is the duty of followers to do whatever they can to prolong and protect their lives, even if it means breaking other religious injunctions.

2. Does Judaism prescribe a particular type of dress for men or women?

Reform and Liberal Jews are likely to wear clothing particular to their culture, not religion. Women may choose to cover their hair while praying, and men may wear a *kippah* or *yamulkah* (skullcap).

Some Orthodox Jews wear formalized clothing; for example, men may choose to wear a hat and/or religious undergarment at all times. Some men grow *peyot* (sidelocks) and maintain long beards. Orthodox women will likely cover their heads when leaving their homes, as well as their arms and legs. In order to accommodate modesty requirements, hospitals should offer long hospital gowns that do not open in the back and which cover the arms. Patients may also resist removal of their head coverings.

3. Are there any prayer or ritual observances that are likely to occur during the patient's stay?

Observant Jews will pray formally three times during the day: in the morning, at noon, and in the evening. Judaism teaches that both males and females should cover their heads during prayer. Men will wear a skullcap while women often wear a headscarf. A quiet room should be provided for prayer when possible.

Some Jews wear *tefillin* during prayer; tefillin are small black cubes that are tied to the dominant arm and forehead to remind the wearer that his thoughts and actions are guided by G-d. Men may also choose to wear a prayer shawl (*tallit*). If patients have trouble putting on the tefillin or tallit, assistance should be offered.

For many Jews, the Sabbath is the most important ongoing ritual. The Jewish Sabbath begins at sunset on Friday and lasts until after sunset on Saturday. Sabbath is meant to be a day of rest, and there are many injunctions against activities considered "work." Depending on the patient's degree of observance, possible conflicts with hospital care include injunctions against turning lights on or off, pressing buttons (e.g., to summon a nurse), signing one's name, and preparing medication (e.g., drawing up insulin).

Additionally, some observant Jews do not drive on the Sabbath, leading to difficulty with a Saturday discharge. If possible, visiting hours should be extended on Saturdays for patients who strictly observe the Sabbath, and may receive visitors later in the day when the Sabbath has ended. As a general rule, operations and procedures should be avoided on the Sabbath. Sabbath observers may also wish to light candles to mark its start and finish; this should be accommodated if possible. If lighting a fire is prohibited, you may instead offer electric candelabras.

4. Does Judaism have hygiene or washing requirements?

Orthodox Jews will likely cleanse themselves before prayer, and before and after eating. If they are unable to access running water, a bowl and jug of water should be offered.

Some Orthodox Jews will choose not to bathe or shower during major festivals or the Sabbath. Some men also prefer to be bearded.

5. Are there any dietary restrictions?

Food that is permissible according to Jewish law is called *kosher*. Kosher food is that which G-d has specifically stated is permissible. Guidelines include:

- Fish must have both scales and fins (which *excludes* shellfish).

- Cows, sheep, goats, and most poultry are permissible; pigs and rabbits are not.

- Permissible animals must be butchered and prepared in a kosher way (e.g., gelatin).

- Fruits and vegetables must be washed and free from insects.

- Milk and its derivatives cannot be eaten in combination with meat and its derivatives.

Offer observant patients sealed packets of food that are branded as kosher. If this is not possible, a vegetarian diet is acceptable as long as it meets cleanliness requirements. You may also allow the patient's friends and family to bring kosher food. This is especially important for many Orthodox Jews, who will not eat food prepared in a non-kosher kitchen unless produced under Rabbinic supervision.

Patients may choose to fast on certain holidays, particularly Yom Kippur and *Tisha B'Av*. These fasts last for 25 hours, beginning before sunset on the eve of the holiday and ending after nightfall the next day. If fasting threatens one's health, it is permissible to abstain. Children under the age of nine and women in labor or within three days postpartum are *not* permitted to fast. Observant Jews with other health problems may wish to consult a rabbi for advice if they feel uncomfortable breaking the fast for medical reasons.

6. Are there any medications, treatments, or procedures that Jews cannot accept?

Jewish patients that keep a kosher diet will only accept medication that is also kosher. This *excludes* medications or surgical procedures that involve pig or horse derivatives (e.g., pork-based insulin, gelatin, and porcine replacement heart valves). Reform and Liberal Jews are more likely to accept non-kosher medication.

If a patient is fasting for religious reasons, s/he will likely accept injections but may resist oral medications.

Patients from very Orthodox communities may resist any medical treatment, including routine blood tests, during the Sabbath or holidays, unless absolutely necessary.

7. Can Jewish patients see providers of the opposite sex?

Many Jews will not object to receiving medical care from providers of the opposite sex. However, those from more Orthodox communities may feel uncomfortable with this, and a provider of the same sex should be offered. If this is not possible, the patient may feel more comfortable if a family member or second staff member of the same sex is present in the room.

8. Can Jews donate organs or accept donor organs?

There is no universal consensus in Judaism on organ donation and acceptance. Generally, it is permissible if necessary to save a life.

Organ removal from a living person is generally permissible if the organs are being used immediately and their removal does not compromise the future health of the donor.

Organ removal from the deceased requires some sensitivity. Organs are not to be harvested until the patient is deceased according to religious law (see question #13), and should not be placed in storage without the family's consent.

9. Should I consult anyone other than the patient when seeking informed consent or other patient decisions?

As a general rule, patients make health care decisions individually. However, some may wish to have members of their faith communities and/or a rabbi talk through a decision with them.

10. What are Judaism's views on reproductive health and family planning? Are contraceptives okay? What about abortion? Voluntary sterilization?

Generally, termination of a pregnancy is permissible if the mother's life is in danger. However, there is some disagreement amongst the branches of Judaism.

Traditionally, a Jewish woman is considered unclean until seven days after her menstrual flow ceases. Thus, observant Jewish women may wish to delay gynecological examinations until this period has passed.

Views on reproductive health and family vary according to denomination. Reform and Liberal Jewish communities are often willing to accept contraceptives. However, Orthodox Jews are likely to rely on the rhythm method or an oral contraceptive; the use of condoms is controversial.

Artificial insemination is generally permitted by all branches of Judaism.

Voluntary sterilization is generally impermissible.

11. Are there particular beliefs or rituals concerning pregnancy and birth? What about postpartum women? What about women who have miscarried?

Orthodox Jewish women are likely to be uncomfortable with male attendants in prenatal examinations and during labor. Orthodox Jewish men may choose to be present during both, but will likely adhere to strict cleanliness rituals; they may not touch their wives or pass objects directly to them.

Boys are usually circumcised eight days after birth if their health allows. Circumcisions are viewed as religious rituals rather than medical procedures, since circumcision initiates the baby boy into the Covenant between G-d and the Jewish people. Circumcisions are normally performed outside the hospital by a *mohel* (a man who is specially trained and medically certified in ritual circumcision). If the circumcision must be performed in the hospital, the family should be given a quiet room in which to perform the ritual.

Jewish tradition dictates that the mother is unclean (in *niddah*) for seven days after the birth of a boy and for fourteen days after a daughter's birth. Afterward, the mother may immerse herself in a ritual cleansing bath (*mikveh*).

If miscarriage occurs, parents will likely wish to bury the child intact so no hair should be removed. However, the placenta may be discarded. In case of either a stillbirth or miscarriage, a quiet room should be offered to friends and families for mourning.

Judaism teaches that a fetus is alive after 40 days of gestation. Thus, miscarriages after this period will be handled in the same way as an adult's death (see question #13).

12. Are there important end-of-life rituals or beliefs?

Judaism teaches that people have a responsibility to accept medical treatment if it will save their lives. If a treatment is believed to extend life or it holds a possibility of recovery, some Jews believe it is their duty to accept it. This is a topic of extreme sensitivity and variance of belief.

Many Reform and Liberal Jews will accept brain death as the moment of death. However, more Orthodox Jews may follow the traditional definition of death found in Jewish law: a body without breath or heartbeat for a period of time, making resuscitation impossible. If organ donation has been agreed to, the possible conflict between the time the organs must be removed and the moment of death should be discussed with the patient, family, and a rabbi.

Depending on the patient's denomination, the patient may wish to have a rabbi hear his/her confession (*vidui*) and pray with him/her before death. In particular, the patient may wish to hear special psalms or prayer; Judaism teaches that the holiest prayer, the *shema*, is the last thing a person should hear before dying. Privacy and quiet should be provided.

Patients will likely be visited by friends and family. Visitors may wish to pray with the patient and recite special parts of scriptures.

13. What should be done with the body after death?

As a general rule, the body should not be touched until 8 minutes after death. Typically, the body is not left alone, and family members may wish to stay in the room until the body is removed. It is generally considered insulting to eat, drink, laugh, or talk in front of the corpse.

Even if no family members are with the patient when s/he dies, the body should *not* be left alone or in the dark before burial if possible. A candle should be lit and placed near the head of the body; if this is not permissible, a light should be turned and left on.

Often, family members will wish to close the eyes and mouth and straighten the limbs. If no family member is present, this should be done by the provider. However, the body should be touched as little as possible.

There are local Jewish burial societies (called the *chevra kaddisha*) who care for the deceased. These volunteers wash the body and dress it in a special shroud; this should *not* be done by a health care provider unless requested by the family. Volunteers from the burial societies may stay with the body to recite psalms constantly until the burial service.

Many Jews prefer to bury their dead within 24 hours of death when possible.

For Sabbath-observant Jews, patients who die on Fridays should not be moved to the mortuary until Saturday night, when those preparing the body for burial can collect it. It should be left in a lit area at all times. This rule may also apply on certain Jewish holidays.

Postmortems are accepted if required by law. Whether they are accepted when not required varies based on both the patient's individual beliefs and his/her denomination.

· · · ·

Judaism: Intersections with Health Care

Judaism is a religion that dates back approximately 4,000 years. Throughout the religion's history, it has placed a strong emphasis on the sanctity of human life, making the preserving and prolonging of life a religious duty. This often leads to a complementary relationship between Western medicine and Jewish beliefs. However, some Jewish denominations place a strong emphasis on traditional Jewish laws set forth thousands of years ago, leading to potential conflicts with modern medical practices.

Quick answers for what to do when such a conflict arises may be found in the FAQ. For more in-depth explanations, consult the appropriate section below.

CAUSES OF ILLNESS & HEALING RITUALS

Judaism strikes a balance between recognizing purely medical explanations for illness and viewing illness as part of a divine plan. The Talmud, one of the main sources of Jewish law, emphasizes the sanctity of human life; it is the duty of followers to do whatever they can to prolong and protect their lives even if this means breaking other religious injunctions.

Generally, though there is a high value given to Western medical treatment, G-d is still recognized as the ultimate healer. Therefore, many Jews will pray for their health during times of illness. Visitation and helping the sick are also highly valued, and considered a *mitzvah* (a Jewish commandment).

DRESS & MODESTY

Dress requirements differ significantly between the Reform and Liberal Jewish traditions on one hand and the Orthodox tradition on the other.

Reform and Liberal Jews are likely to wear clothing particular to their culture, not religion. Women may choose to cover their hair while praying, and men may wear a kippah or yarmulke (skullcap). This is done in observance of the teachings of the *Mishneh Torah*, a code of Jewish law written by the Jewish leader and philosopher Maimonides in the 12th century. Maimonides taught that covering one's hair during prayer was a rule given by Moses and is, thus, religiously mandatory.

Tzni'ut is a Hebrew word meaning "modesty" that is used to describe modesty as both a character trait and as a reference to a group of Jewish religious laws on modesty. These laws are most influential in Orthodox Judaism. In observance of tzni'ut, some Orthodox Jews wear formalized clothing; for example, men may choose to wear a hat, kippah, and/or religious undergarment at all times. Some men grow peyot (sidelocks) and maintain long beards in observance of verses 17 through 26 of the Book of Leviticus (also known as the *Holiness Code)*, which forbids the "shaving of the corners of the head" and the "marring" of the "corners of the beard." Orthodox women will likely cover their heads when leaving their homes, as well as their arms and legs; many wear wigs outside the house.

In order to accommodate modesty requirements, hospitals should offer long hospital gowns that do not open in the back and which cover the arms. Patients may also resist removal of their head coverings; tension may be eased if the patient is offered an alternative head covering, such as a scrub cap.

PRAYER & RITUAL OBSERVANCES

Observant Jews will pray formally three times during the day: in the morning, at noon and in the evening. Judaism teaches that both males and females should cover their heads during prayer. This demonstrates one's recognition that G-d is above humankind, acceptance of Jewish commandments, and identification as a member of the Jewish community. Men will wear a skullcap, while women often wear a headscarf. A quiet room should be provided for prayer when possible.

Some Jews wear tefillin during prayer; tefillin are small black cubes that are tied to the dominant arm and forehead to remind the wearer that his thoughts and actions are guided by G-d. Men may also choose to wear a prayer shawl (tallit). The most important parts of the tallit are the twined and knotted fringes on its four corners, called *tzitzit*; the wearing of tzitzit is a religious requirement found in the Torah. If patients have trouble putting on the tefillin or tallit, assistance should be offered.

For many Jews, the Sabbath is the most important ongoing ritual. The Jewish Sabbath begins at sunset on Friday and lasts until after sunset on Saturday. The Sabbath is a celebration of G-d's creation of the world and day of rest afterwards; it is a time to celebrate the family and Jewish community.

Sabbath is meant to be a day of rest, and there are many injunctions against activities considered "work." For observant Jews, possible conflicts with hospital care include injunctions against turning lights on or off, pressing buttons (e.g., to summon a nurse), signing one's name, and preparing medication (e.g., drawing up insulin). It is important for health care providers to discuss Sabbath practices with Jewish patients to find out what activities they will not feel comfortable doing and may need assistance with.

Some observant Jews do not drive on the Sabbath, which can create difficulty with a Saturday discharge. In addition, if possible, visiting hours should be extended on Saturdays for patients who strictly observe the Sabbath and may receive visitors later in the day when the Sabbath has ended.

As a general rule, operations and procedures should be avoided on the Sabbath. Observers may also wish to light candles to mark its start and finish; this should be accommodated if possible. If lighting a fire is prohibited, you may instead offer electric candelabras.

Many Jews of all denominations go to their local synagogue for community prayer and Torah readings on the Sabbath. It is an important time for spiritual and community building. If a patient is unable to attend his/her synagogue, family members and/or a rabbi might visit the patient.

HYGIENE & WASHING REQUIREMENTS

Orthodox Jews will likely cleanse themselves before prayer and before and after eating, in observance of rituals laid down in the Torah. If they are unable to access running water, a bowl and jug of water and assistance with washing should be offered. Observant Jews will wish to pray three times a day: in the morning, around noon, and in the evening, and may want to wash before each of these. While cleansing rituals are being performed, privacy should be given.

Some Orthodox Jews will choose not to bathe or shower during major festivals or the Sabbath. Some men also prefer to be bearded.

DIETARY REQUIREMENTS

Food that is permissible according to Jewish law is called kosher. Kosher food is that which G-d has specifically stated is permissible. The basic division of food into kosher and non-kosher can be found in the Torah's Book of Leviticus and Deuteronomy, while the detail of what constitutes kosher versus non-kosher food was established in Jewish oral laws (specifically, the Mishnah Torah and the Talmud).

Guidelines include:

- Fish must have both scales and fins (which *excludes* shellfish).

- Cows, sheep, goats and most poultry are permissible; pigs and rabbits are not.

- Permissible animals must be butchered and prepared in a kosher way.

- Fruits and vegetables must be washed and free from insects.

- Milk and its derivatives cannot be eaten in combination with meat and its derivatives (e.g., gelatin).

In order to keep milk and meat completely separate, many people leave a gap of several hours between eating the two. The time which must elapse varies among Jews from different traditions and national origins, and can range from 20 minutes (typically, the time that must elapse after consumption of dairy) to 6 hours (the maximum time that must elapse after consumption of meat). Among Orthodox Jews, common waiting periods post-meat are 3 hours, 5 hours and 1 minute, and 6 hours.

In addition to the value of following Jewish law, there are other theological reasons for maintaining a kosher diet. Judaism teaches that following a law given by G-d helps one to concentrate the mind on G-d's will and one's duty to G-d. It is a demonstration of one's commitment to the faith and helps provide a sense of connection to others who follow the same commandments. Thus, it helps maintain one's identity as a member of the Jewish community. Additionally, kosher rules help to ensure that animals are treated with greater kindness. Maintaining a kosher diet is also believed to keep one physically healthier.

Offer observant patients sealed packets of food that are branded as kosher. If this is not possible, a vegetarian diet is acceptable as long as it meets cleanliness requirements. If possible, allow the patient's friends and family to bring kosher food; this is especially important for many Orthodox Jews, who will not eat food prepared in a non-kosher kitchen unless produced under rabbinic supervision.

Patients may choose to fast from both food and liquid on certain holidays, particularly Yom Kippur and Tisha B'Av. These fasts last for 25 hours, beginning before sunset on the eve of the holiday and ending after nightfall the next day. Yom Kippur is the Jewish Day of Atonement; it is the holiest and most solemn day of the Jewish calendar; in addition to fasting, most or all of the day is usually spent in worship and contemplation. Tisha B'Av is a day of solemn fasting in remembrance of the destruction of the first and second temples in Jerusalem.

For those observing fasts on these two holidays, it is important to note that there are exceptions made for illness. If fasting threatens one's health, it is permissible to abstain. Feeding a patient through a nasogastric tube or with IV is not legally considered eating according to Jewish law. Additionally, children under the age of nine and women in labor or within three days postpartum are *not* permitted to fast. Observant Jews with other health problems may wish to consult a rabbi for advice if they feel uncomfortable breaking the fast for medical reasons.

MEDICATION, TREATMENT, AND PROCEDURE RESTRICTIONS
Jewish patients who keep a kosher diet (see Dietary Requirements) may only accept medication that is also kosher. This will *exclude* medications or surgical procedures that involve pig or horse derivatives (e.g., pork-based insulin, gelatin, and porcine replacement heart valves). Reform and Liberal Jews are more likely to accept non-kosher medication.

If a patient is fasting for religious reasons, either during the Sabbath or a religious holiday, s/he will likely accept injections but may resist oral medications. Patients from very Orthodox communities may resist any medical treatment, including routine blood tests, during the Sabbath or holidays unless absolutely necessary.

There is, however, a provision within Jewish law that stipulates that the duty to save life overrules any other considerations; thus the restriction on non-kosher medicines may be broken if the patient is in immediate danger of death, or if the non-kosher treatment is the only one available. Given the sensitivity of this topic, practitioners are encouraged to involve a rabbi in the conversation if this issue arises.

GENDER & MODESTY

Tzni'ut is a Hebrew word meaning "modesty" that is used to describe modesty as both a character trait and as a reference to a group of Jewish religious laws on modesty.

These laws are most influential in Orthodox Judaism, which teaches that men and women are not allowed to touch one another unless they are married; nor are they allowed to enter into a secluded room or a private area for more than a few seconds. Thus, while most Jews will not object to receiving medical care from providers of the opposite sex, those from more Orthodox communities are likely to feel uncomfortable with this. For these patients, a provider of the same sex should be offered. If this is not possible, the patient may feel more comfortable if a family member or even another staff person is present in the room, so that the doctor and patient are not alone together.

ORGAN DONATION

There is no universal consensus in Judaism on organ donation and acceptance. Generally, it is permissible if necessary to save a life.

Organ removal from a living person is generally permissible if the organs are being used immediately and their removal does not compromise the future health of the donor.

Organ removal from the deceased requires some sensitivity. Organs are not to be harvested until the patient is deceased according to religious law (see End of Life), and should not be placed in storage without the family's consent.

INFORMED CONSENT & PATIENT DECISION MAKING

As a general rule, patients make health care decisions individually. However, some may wish to have members of their faith communities and/or a rabbi talk through a decision with them.

REPRODUCTIVE HEALTH & FAMILY PLANNING

Traditionally, Jewish women are considered unclean for seven days after their menstrual flows cease; this state of uncleanliness is called niddah. This tradition stems from the Torah, which states that a menstruating woman should be separated from other people for seven days because she is not "ritually pure". According to this regulation, any man who has sexual intercourse with a woman in niddah is also considered ritually impure.

The extent to which this biblical law is followed in modern Judaism varies according to the denomination. Conservative Judaism teaches that adherents should refrain from sexual relations during this time; however, its rule for the length of niddah differs from that of Orthodox Judaism. Conservative Judaism teaches that niddah lasts for a total of seven days, beginning with the first day of menstruation. In contrast, Orthodox Judaism teaches that niddah lasts for seven days following the *last* day of menstruation. In addition to refraining from sexual activity during this time, many Orthodox Jewish women ritually wash themselves at the end of this period. Jewish women observing niddah may wish to delay gynecological examinations until this period has passed.

Views on reproductive health and family vary according to denomination. Followers of Reform and Liberal Judaism are often willing to accept contraceptives. However, Orthodox Jews are likely to rely on the rhythm method or an oral contraceptive; the use of condoms is controversial due to a prohibition in Jewish law against the "spilling of seed." Additionally, the Torah compels Jews to go forth and multiply; some Jews interpret this as barring all sex that is non-procreative. Artificial insemination is generally permitted.

Voluntary sterilization is generally impermissible, as it is believed to be a violation of G-d's plan for humans to procreate; Orthodox Jewish patients are more likely to uphold this teaching. However, if sterilization is a medical necessity, Jewish law teaches that it must be carried out given the high value of human life.

In Jewish law, an unborn fetus is regarded as part of the mother's body and is considered human at 40 days' gestation. However, it is not considered a full-fledged human being until labor has begun. While Judaism holds that all life is of infinite value, it also holds that the life of a human who has been born takes precedence over that of a human still in the womb. Accordingly, the life of the mother takes precedence over that of the fetus and termination of a pregnancy is permissible if the mother's life is in danger. Abortion is generally *not* permissible on the grounds of genetic imperfections in the fetus. If there is a question over what constitutes a threat to the life of a mother, Judaism teaches that a rabbi trained in Jewish law should be consulted.

PREGNANCY & BIRTH

Orthodox Jewish women are likely to be uncomfortable with male attendants in prenatal examinations and during labor. Orthodox Jewish men may choose to be present during both, but will likely adhere to strict cleanliness rituals; they may not touch their wives or pass objects directly to them due to a law that physical contact should not be made between the couple once there has been any blood loss by the woman.

If a planned induction or elective cesarean is necessary, parents who strictly observe the Sabbath may prefer to avoid having these procedures performed during the Sabbath.

Boys are usually circumcised eight days after birth if their health allows; this ceremony is called *Brit Milah*. Circumcisions are viewed as religious rituals rather than medical procedures, since the circumcision ritual is what initiates the baby boy into the Covenant between G-d and the Jewish people.

Circumcisions are normally performed outside the hospital by a mohel (a man trained and medically certified in ritual circumcision). If the circumcision must be performed in the hospital, the family should be given a quiet room in which to perform the ritual. A male baby is traditionally named on the day of his circumcision, whereas a girl's name is traditionally announced by her father in the synagogue at the first Torah reading following birth.

Jewish tradition dictates that the mother is unclean (in niddah) for seven days after the birth of a boy and for 14 days after a daughter's birth. During this period, she is to refrain from sexual intercourse. After this period has passed, she may immerse herself in a ritual cleansing bath (mikveh); this is generally done only by Orthodox Jewish women, although many Conservative Jewish women will also abstain from sexual activity during this period.

If a miscarriage occurs, parents will likely wish to bury the child intact, although the placenta may be discarded. In case of either a stillbirth or miscarriage, a quiet room should be offered to friends and families for mourning.

Judaism teaches that a fetus is alive after 40 days of gestation. Thus, miscarriages occurring after this period will be handled in the same way as an adult's death (see question #13).

END OF LIFE

Judaism teaches that people have a responsibility to accept medical treatment if it will save their lives. If a treatment is believed to extend life or it holds a possibility of recovery, some Jews believe it is their duty to accept it. This is a topic of extreme sensitivity and variance of belief, and opinion is divided about whether or not treatment artificially prolonging life is required or not. It is strongly suggested that a rabbi who is skilled in Jewish medical ethics be brought into the conversation if this is an issue with the patient.

Many Reform and Liberal Jews will accept brain death as the moment of death. However, more Orthodox Jews may follow the traditional definition of death found in Jewish law: a body without breath or heartbeat for a period of time making resuscitation impossible. If organ donation has been agreed to, the possible conflict between the time the organs must be removed and the moment of death should be discussed with the patient, family, and a rabbi.

Depending on the patient's denomination, they may wish to have a rabbi hear their confession (vidui) and pray with them before death. In particular, they may wish to hear special psalms or prayer; Judaism teaches that the holiest prayer, the shema, is the last thing a person should hear before dying. Privacy and quiet should be provided.

Patients will likely be visited by friends and family. Visitors may wish to pray with the patient and recite special parts of scriptures.

As a general rule, the body should not be touched until 8 minutes after death. Typically, the body is not left alone, and family members may wish to stay in the room until the body is removed. It is generally considered insulting to eat, drink, laugh, or talk in front of the corpse.

Even if no family members are with the patient when s/he dies, the body should not be left alone or in the dark before burial if possible; the body is considered to be G-d's property and must be treated with extreme respect. A lit candle should be placed near the head of the body; if this is not permissible, a light should be turned and left on. Often, family members will wish to close the eyes and mouth and straighten the limbs. If no family member is present, this should be done by the provider, but the body should be touched as little as possible.

There are local Jewish burial societies called the chevra kaddisha who care for the deceased. They are special members of the Jewish community designated to carry out this task so that others need not, because of a belief that bodies are unclean once life has ceased. These volunteers wash the body and dress it in a special shroud; this should *not* be done by a health care provider unless requested by the family. Volunteers from the burial societies may stay with the body to recite psalms constantly until the burial service. Women attend to the bodies of women and children, while men attend to the bodies of men.

Members of the chevra kaddisha traditionally perform their duties anonymously so that the bereaved family does not feel under any obligation to them. They will collect the body from the hospital as soon as possible after death to ensure a quicker burial. Many Jews prefer to bury their dead within 24 hours of death when possible. In the United States, it is common for these burial societies to be organized by each synagogue, although not every synagogue has one.

For Sabbath-observant Jews, patients who die on Fridays should not be moved to the mortuary until Saturday night, when those preparing the body for burial can collect it. It should be left in a lit area at all times. This rule may also apply on certain Jewish holidays.

During the seven days following the burial, Orthodox families sit *Shiva*. During this time, the deceased's immediate family stays at home and is visited and comforted by family, friends, and acquaintances. In some communities, visitors may bring food. Traditionally, male relatives recite *Kaddish*, the prayer for the dead, in the synagogue. Formal mourning is suspended on the Sabbath.

Postmortems are accepted if required by law. Whether they are accepted when not required varies based on both the patient's individual beliefs and his/her denomination.

Orthodox Jews are unlikely to consent unless it is required by law because it is considered to be a desecration of the body; many believe that when the Messiah comes, the dead will be revived, making it necessary for bodies to be buried intact. For those following this tradition, even a legally required postmortem will likely cause distress. In this case, relatives must be approached with great sensitivity and be assured that the body is complete after the postmortem.

Autopsies should be done as quickly as possible following death, since many families will want to bury the deceased within 24 hours of death. Those performing a postmortem should not place the body face down, and should keep the body covered as much as possible.

FOR MORE READING: JUDAISM

Jakobovits I. Judaism and medicine. In: Goodacre D, ed. *World Religions and Medicine*. 2nd ed. Oxford, UK: Institute of Religion and Medicine. 1983: 33–42.

Leavitt R. Cultural considerations for Jewish clients. In: Lattanzi JB, Purnell LD, eds. *Developing Cultural Competence in Physical Therapy Practice*. Philadelphia, PA: JA Davis. 2006: 276–90.

Leininger M. Jewish Americans and Russian Jews culture care. In: Leininger M, McFarland MR, eds. *Transcultural Nursing: Concepts, Theories, Research and Practice*. 3rd ed. New York, NY: McGraw-Hill. 2002: 465–75.

Sager RSG. Eye on religion: The reflective physician and the Jewish patient. *Southern Med J*. 2006; 99[10]: 1186–87.

Schott J, Henley A. Judaism. In: Schott J, Henley A, eds. *Culture, Religion and Childbearing in a Multiracial Society*. Oxford, UK: Butterworth-Heinemann. 1996: 329–38.

2. Christianity

Overview FAQ

1. When, where, and how did Christianity originate?

Christianity emerged during the first century CE in what is present-day Israel, and is based on the belief that Jesus of Nazareth was the *Messiah* (the "anointed one") awaited by the Jewish people as their redeemer.

Jesus' teachings attracted many Jewish followers during his lifetime. After his crucifixion at the hands of the Roman Empire, his followers, convinced of his divinity, formed communities. Originally sects of Judaism, these communities sought and accepted large numbers of believers and developed into a separate religion over several centuries, now recognized as Christianity.

2. Does Christianity have sacred texts? What are they called?

The Bible is the sacred text for Christians. It has two main parts: the Old Testament (which is almost the same as Judaism's Hebrew Bible, although arranged in a different order) and the New Testament. The New Testament consists of the Gospels, which give accounts of Jesus' life, death, resurrection, and teachings; the Epistles (formal letters) written by early Christian leaders to nascent church communities on theology; and the Book of Revelation, which gives a vision of the end times.

Most Christians believe that the Bible was written by human authors who were divinely inspired to record God's revelations. Some Christians believe that it is the literal, inerrant word of God.

3. What are the core beliefs of Christianity?

Christianity teaches that there is one God, who is manifest in three forms, together making up a Holy Trinity: the Father (Creator), the Son (Redeemer), and the Holy Spirit (Sustainer).

Most Christians believe that Jesus Christ is the incarnation of the second component of the Trinity. Christianity teaches that Jesus was conceived by the Holy Spirit but born to a human woman (the Virgin Mary); thus, Jesus was both fully human and fully divine. Jesus Christ's teachings provide guidance to Christians for living a moral life. Christianity also teaches that Jesus' death and resurrection paved the way for humans to overcome sin and be reconciled to God. Thus, Jesus Christ offers salvation and the promise of eternal life, which is viewed as a gift from God.

4. What are the core practices of Christianity?

Most Christians consider prayer to be a cornerstone of their faith. Christianity teaches that prayer allows the believer to communicate directly with God. Additionally, Catholics may choose to pray with Saints. Saints are not believed to be gods themselves, but rather are guardians over different areas of life, and function as prayer intermediaries. Prayer may be done in private or communally, depending on the individual, denomination, or culture. Public prayer most often occurs on the Sabbath, usually a Sunday, when most Christian traditions hold worship services (the Seventh-day Adventist community observes the Sabbath on Saturdays, while Jehovah's Witnesses do not observe a Sabbath at all). Sunday worship services vary according to denomination, but may include singing, a message delivered by clergy (called a sermon or homily), readings from the Bible, communal prayer, confession of sins, an offering, and *Communion* (also called the *Eucharist*).

Communion is a ritual re-creating Jesus' final meal with his followers. During that meal, called the *Last Supper*, Jesus offered his closest disciples bread and wine to symbolize his body and blood. The communion ritual commemorates this meal. Some denominations believe that after the wine and bread are blessed, they are transfigured into Jesus Christ's actual body and blood. Others believe the bread and wine are symbolic of Jesus' sacrifice.

Communion is considered a *sacrament* by many denominations. Sacraments are ritual acts through which Christians receive divine grace. The number and type of sacraments differ according to denomination. Other sacraments may include: baptism (which symbolizes a rebirth into the faith); confirmation (membership into the church); repentance; marriage; anointing of the sick; and holy orders (when clergy are ordained).

5. What are Christianity's important holidays? How are they celebrated?

The most important holiday for Christians is Easter, which is a commemoration of the Resurrection of Jesus Christ. On this day, Christians celebrate the overcoming of sin and death. Many Christians attend church in the morning and spend the day in festive celebration with their families. The 40 days preceding Easter are called Lent. Lent is a period of penitence and self-examination for many Christians, some of whom fast or observe dietary restrictions during this period.

Christmas, which celebrates the birth of Jesus Christ, is another important day for Christians. The traditions surrounding Christmas vary by denomination and region, but Christians worldwide traditionally attend church on either Christmas day or on Christmas Eve. The holiday is normally spent with family, and may include communal meals or gift exchanges. Christmas is a day of goodwill, compassion, and peace.

Eastern Orthodox denominations use the Julian calendar; thus holy days like Easter and Christmas will fall on different dates than those observed by Catholic, Protestant, and other Christian denominations.

6. How many adherents of Christianity are there in the United States? Are they located in a particular region?

Christianity is the predominant religion in the United States. Approximately 80% of the population considers itself Christian, and adherents are dispersed geographically.

The highest concentration of Christians can be found in the South, but substantial populations are found nationwide.

7. What are the main sects or denominations within Christianity?

The three largest groupings of Christianity are: Eastern Orthodox, Roman Catholic, and Protestant, with many smaller denominations falling within these branches.

- The **Eastern Orthodox** Church considers itself to be the historical, unbroken continuation of the original Christian community established by Jesus Christ. It teaches that the purpose of the Christian life is to attain a mystical union with God (*theosis*). There are 14 branches of the Church, including the Ecumenical Patriarchate of Constantinople, and the Greek, Russian, Serbian, Romanian, Bulgarian, Georgian, and Cypriot Orthodox churches, all headed by their own leaders; most recognize the Ecumenical Patriarch of Constantinople as the most senior leader.

    The Eastern Orthodox Church is highly ritualized. The services are composed nearly entirely of chanting, with incense and icons playing an important role. Observant Orthodox Christians may spend one-half of the year fasting at various levels of strictness, while the sacraments form the basis of the practicing of the faith.

- The **Roman Catholic** Church also considers itself to be the historical, unbroken continuation of the original Christian community established by Jesus Christ. The Catholic Church is divided into territories (called dioceses), each headed by a bishop. At the top of this hierarchy sits the Bishop of Rome, commonly known as the Pope, who is the highest human authority on faith, morals, and church governance. In addition to the moral guidelines provided in the Bible, Catholics have developed a system of canon law that outlines the church's teachings on theology. As in the Eastern Orthodox Church, sacraments play an important role in the lives of adherents.

- **Protestantism** emerged in the 16th century and was initially a movement against the institution and hierarchy of the Catholic church. Today, the Protestant tradition embraces a wide variety of denominations, including: Anglican/Episcopalian, Baptist, Lutheran, Methodist, Pentecostal, Presbyterian, Society of Friends (Quakers), and United Church of Christ. However, many Protestants do not formally affiliate with a single denomination and may move between them with relative ease.

    Protestant churches are generally less hierarchical than their Eastern Orthodox and Roman Catholic counterparts. Most Protestants observe only two sacraments: baptism and communion. Often, Protestant churches emphasize the importance of reading the Bible both individually and communally and stress direct communication with God.

Some Protestants self-identify as evangelical. Broadly speaking, the beliefs of evangelicals include a responsibility to preaching and teaching the good news found in the scriptures in such a way as to encourage conversion to the faith. Some do this by living their lives in accordance with their beliefs, while others seek to engage people on the issue more directly.

In addition, there are several branches of Christianity in the United States that have substantive theological differences with Eastern Orthodox, Catholic, and Protestant denominations. They include the following:

- The **Church of Jesus Christ of Latter Day Saints** emerged in the United States in the early 19th century with Joseph Smith, who wrote the Book of Mormon after receiving divine revelation. Mormons have a strong missionary ministry and are thus found worldwide. However, their center is in Salt Lake City, Utah. Most Mormons attend church regularly (and, following their participation in prescribed rituals, attend the Temple on special occasions) and follow a strict set of moral guidelines and practices.

- **Christian Science** is a religious teaching that emerged with Mary Baker Eddy's book *Science and Health with Key to the Scriptures*, first published in 1875. Christian Scientists believe in the efficacy of the fundamental healing power of God for the faithful and often refuse medical interventions.

- **Jehovah's Witnesses** are members of a religion that believes itself to be a restored form of first-century Christianity. They believe that contemporary Christianity is corrupted, and dispute the doctrines of the Trinity and the immortality of the soul. Jehovah's Witnesses are perhaps best known for their conviction in the importance of spreading their beliefs to others, primarily through house visits.

- **The Seventh-day Adventist** Church was formally established in 1863, in the United States. Though many of its theological tenets are the same as mainline Protestant churches, Adventists believe that the soul sleeps unconsciously between the death of the body and its resurrection when the Apocalypse arrives. The Church also teaches that judgment of Christian believers has been in progress since 1844. Adventists observe the Sabbath on Saturday, and most consider themselves to be evangelical. The Church emphasizes diet and health and promotes a socially conservative lifestyle.

• • • •

Intersections with Health Care: FAQ

1. Does Christianity have a particular view about what causes illness? Are there illness-related rituals?

Most Christians accept Western medical explanations for causes of illness.

Adherents of many Christian denominations use prayer in some way during times of illness. Some believe that prayer can facilitate the healing process and possibly cause a miraculous cure that medical treatment alone could not achieve. Others view prayer as a necessary component of one's overall well-being and mental and spiritual health, but not physical health. It is common for Christian patients to receive visitors who will pray with them for their health.

Some denominations have more specific rituals and beliefs:

- Members of some denominations, particularly Catholics, will want clergy to visit and perform the sacrament of the *anointing of the sick*. During the sacrament, clergy anoint the individual with holy oil or water that has been blessed; traditionally, the eyes, ears, nostrils, lips, hands, and feet are anointed. The sacrament may be performed at any time during a hospital stay and is often requested pre-surgery.

- Christian Science teaches that death and disease are illusory and discourages medical treatment in favor of spiritual healing actualized through specific prayers. Christian Scientists who have entered the hospital voluntarily will likely accept only minimal medical treatment and drug therapy. Those who have arrived involuntarily may wish to be released with no treatment.

2. Does Christianity prescribe a particular type of dress for men or women?

There is no prescribed dress code for most Christian denominations, although more conservative sects tend to wear more modest clothing. Particular churches may have their own internal guidelines.

Christians may wear religious jewelry (e.g., a necklace with a pendant of a cross or saint). Some religious jewelry may have been blessed by a spiritual leader and should not be removed without consent. Additionally, Christians may bring a rosary (prayer beads), small icons (a religious painting or statue), or a vessel of holy water into the hospital with them. These should be handled with great respect.

Members of the Church of Jesus Christ of Latter-Day Saints (Mormons) may wear a type of underclothing called simply a *garment*, which represents their promises to God. The garment may be removed for care, although some older patients may resist its removal.

3. Are there any prayer or ritual observances that are likely to occur during the patient's stay?

The most common ritual observances health care providers may encounter are baptism and communion. Depending on the denomination, baptism can entail anything from a sprinkle of water on a patient's head to total immersion in water. This ceremony marks a Christian's birth into the faith. Some denominations teach that infants should be baptized at birth, while others believe that baptism should be held off until a person is old enough to choose the faith for him or herself. If a Christian patient was not baptized at birth, s/he may wish to be baptized in the hospital if death is imminent. Additionally, Christian parents may wish to have a baby baptized in the hospital if the child is very ill because they fear that the baby will not go to heaven if s/he is not baptized; this can be a cause of great distress for parents. Baptisms are traditionally performed by ordained clergy.

Communion (also called the Eucharist) is a key ritual for many Christians and involves consuming bread and wine (or juice) that has been blessed and distributed by clergy. Communion may be taken on a denomination's Sabbath, on holidays, or at any time clergy deem it appropriate. Roman Catholics may wish to confess to a priest and fast for an hour before receiving communion.

Additionally, patients may wish to read the Bible and/or pray, either individually or with other Christians. Patients may appreciate a separate room in which to pray.

Sunday is the traditional day of worship for the majority of Christian denominations (some observe the Sabbath on Saturday, notably Seventh-day Adventists). If a patient is unable to attend a formal service on his/her Sabbath, s/he may receive special visitations from family and/or spiritual leaders. Seventh-day Adventists may refuse treatment on Friday evenings and Saturdays as part of their observance.

Icons are extremely important in religious practice for Orthodox Christians. Accordingly, most will bring icons with them to the hospital. Patient consent is necessary before handling these objects.

4. Does Christianity have hygiene or washing requirements?

Generally, there are no hygiene or washing requirements for Christian patients.

5. Are there any dietary restrictions?

Some Roman Catholics may abstain from eating meat on Fridays and others may wish to fast before receiving Communion.

Strict Orthodox Christians observe a number of fasting times throughout the year, including fasting on Wednesdays and Fridays, and abstaining from meat and dairy products. Those with health problems are not expected to fast.

Mormons and Seventh-day Adventists typically abstain from anything containing alcohol or caffeine. Some may find them admissible if they are in medications that are a necessary part of treatment.

Many Seventh-day Adventists and Jehovah's Witnesses are vegetarians.

Christians who are opposed to abortion may be extremely reluctant to have any vaccines that are developed from cell lines derived from aborted human fetuses.

6. Are there any medications, treatments, or procedures that Christians cannot accept?

Jehovah's Witnesses typically permit medication and surgical procedures only if they are deemed absolutely medically necessary; in some cases, they may be refused altogether. Jehovah's Witnesses also customarily refuse blood transfusions for both themselves and their children, even in life-threatening situations, due to their belief that a human must not sustain his/her life with another creature's blood. Consequently, they may also refuse any medical treatment that requires the use of blood or blood products, which includes whole blood, red blood cells, white blood cells, platelets, and plasma. Some Jehovah's Witnesses allow auto-transfusion (where the patient's own blood is collected and re-infused) so long as the blood is not stored and is returned immediately to the patient through a continuous circuit. Blood samples may be taken for testing, provided any unused blood is disposed of properly.

Many Seventh-day Adventists will refuse medications that contain alcohol or animal byproducts.

Christian Scientists are likely to refuse all pain medication, choosing instead to heal themselves through specific religious practices. Surgical procedures, amputations, and biopsies are generally forbidden. There are some "mechanical healing tasks" such as setting bones or dressing wounds that are permissible; these should be performed by Christian Science providers if possible. There is a directory of Christian Science nurses in the *Christian Science Journal*.

7. Can Christian patients see providers of the opposite sex?

Most Christians will not object to seeing a provider of the opposite sex. However, more conservative Christians may prefer to see someone of the same sex. Each patient should be asked about their preference.

8. Can Christians donate organs or accept donor organs?

Most Christian denominations have no religious objection to the donation or acceptance of organs. Christian Scientists generally resist all organ, tissue, and body donations; however, each member is free to make his/her own decision.

9. Should I consult anyone other than the patient when seeking informed consent or other patient decisions?

Generally, Christian patients will make decisions individually; however, they may choose to consult members of their faith community.

Jehovah's Witness patients will likely want the Governing Body of their church and/or the elders of their particular community to be involved in health care decisions.

10. What are Christianity's views on reproductive health and family planning? Are contraceptives okay? What about abortion? Voluntary sterilization?

Beliefs on reproductive health and family planning vary according to how conservative a given denomination is. Some Christians view all forms of family planning as acceptable. However, others adamantly oppose all forms of artificial contraception, infertility treatment, and voluntary sterilization, believing that they disrupt God's natural design for procreation. Each individual should be asked about his/her beliefs.

Many Christians are opposed to abortion and, for this reason, may be reluctant to have prenatal testing that may reveal severe birth defects or illnesses for which a prospective parent might want to consider abortion.

11. Are there particular beliefs or rituals concerning pregnancy and birth? What about postpartum women? What about women who have miscarried?

Some Christians may wish to have their babies baptized by clergy shortly after birth if the birth is very premature or the infant is seriously ill. However, only some denominations baptize at birth, so it is important to discuss baptismal preferences with parents.

Since blood transfusions are strictly prohibited for Jehovah's Witnesses, extra care should be taken with their infants to ensure that the infants do not become anemic. A minimum amount of blood should be taken from the baby, and any extra blood from the sample must be disposed of properly.

There is no official religious ceremony that is universally performed for miscarriages, but patients from many denominations may want to have their baby blessed and/or baptized by clergy. The parents may also wish to have a naming service.

12. Are there end-of-life rituals or beliefs I need to know about?

Most Christians will want to be visited by clergy and family prior to death. Visitors will likely pray with the patient and/or read from the Bible.

Some Christians who have not been previously baptized may wish to have this ritual performed. In emergency situations, baptisms may be performed by a hospital chaplain or layperson trusted by the patient.

Others may wish to receive communion, depending on their denomination.

Roman Catholic patients may want to make a final confession to a priest and receive the anointing of the sick (see question #1).

Clergy and family may choose to pray with the patient or read from the Bible.

Direct euthanasia is forbidden by most Christian denominations.

13. What should be done with the body after death?

Most Christians will be comfortable with the ward's normal practice for handling bodies after death.

Christian Scientists prefer that female bodies be handled and prepared for burial by women.

There are no formal religious objections to postmortems in many Christian denominations. A notable exception is Orthodox Christianity, which discourages autopsies, believing that the body must remain intact for Orthodox burial rites.

• • • •

Christianity: Intersections with Health Care

There are over 33,000 distinct denominations of Christianity around the world, with countless understandings of health and illness and widely varying health care related beliefs and practices. Some groups see illness as a natural part of life, while others see it as punishment for past sins. Some allow virtually all medical procedures, while others have strict limits on what types of health care are accessible, and others refuse to access health care at all.

In the face of that tremendous diversity, this manual attempts to do three things:

- Explain the generally accepted Christian understanding of particular topics, where that exists;

- Highlight significant variations with particularly challenging or noteworthy implications for health care practitioners; and

- Create awareness of the range of ways religion impacts care so that providers have a sense of areas in which further inquiry with a patient will be needed.

Quick answers for many questions that arise when caring for a Christian patient may be found in the FAQ. For more in-depth explanations, consult the appropriate section below.

CAUSE OF ILLNESS AND HEALING RITUALS

Many Christians will accept the Western medical explanation offered by their physicians as the cause of their illness, along with the recommended treatment. Some, however, also believe that prayer can facilitate the healing process and possibly cause a miraculous cure that medical treatment alone could not achieve. Others view prayer as a necessary component of one's overall well-being; for them, the aim of prayer is not physical health, but emotional and spiritual health. It is common for Christian patients to receive visitors who will pray with them for their health, including family and friends, clergy, or visitors from their religious congregations.

Members of some denominations, particularly Roman Catholics and some Protestant denominations such as Episcopalians or Anglicans, may want clergy to visit to carry out the sacrament of anointing of the sick. This blessing by a religious leader is believed to aid in the patient's healing. It may be requested and performed at any time during the patient's stay; it is particularly common pre-surgery. In order to bless the patient, clergy may anoint the individual with holy oil or holy water. Traditionally, six parts of the body are anointed: the eyes, ears, nostrils, lips, hands, and feet.

It is important to know that patients from different cultural backgrounds or national origins may have different opinions on when the anointing of the sick is appropriate. In some countries, anointing of the sick is not performed until a patient is very near death. For those patients, asking whether they would like the sacrament or calling in a priest may create a stressful experience and cause them to think that their condition is worse than their practitioners have indicated. Thus, when broaching the topic of anointment, the health care practitioner should explain that in the United States, many people see a clergy member as a routine sacrament ritual, not only during times of serious illness.

Unlike almost all other denominations of Christianity, observant Christian Scientists reject nearly all medical treatment. Christian Science teaches that death and disease are illusory, that the mind has the power to control the physical body, and that physical healing must occur on a spiritual, emotional, and mental level. Believing that Western medical care does not properly address these three levels, Christian Science discourages material medical treatment in favor of spiritual healing, which is actualized through specific prayers. Christian Scientists who have entered the hospital voluntarily will likely accept only minimal medical treatment and drug therapy. Those who have arrived involuntarily may wish to be released with no treatment.

DRESS & MODESTY

There is no prescribed dress code for most Christians, although more conservative denominations of Christianity will tend to wear more modest clothing.

Christians may choose to wear religious jewelry (e.g., a necklace with a pendant of a cross or saint). Some religious jewelry may have been blessed by a spiritual leader and should not be removed without consent. Additionally, Christians may bring a rosary (prayer beads), a small icon (religious painting), or a vessel of holy water into the hospital with them; icons are especially important to followers of Eastern Orthodox Christianity and play a central role in Orthodox worship. These items should not be touched without patient consent, and should then be handled with great respect.

Members of the Church of Jesus Christ of Latter-Day Saints (Mormons) who have committed themselves to the church in a formal ceremony may wear a type of underclothing called a garment, which represents their promises to God and serves as a protector of modesty. The garment may be removed for medical care, although some older patients may resist its removal.

PRAYER & RITUAL OBSERVANCES

The most common ritual observances a health care provider may encounter are *baptism, Holy Communion*, and *confession*.

Baptism is a ceremony in which a person entering a faith tradition is washed as a sign of purification and consecration to God, traditionally performed by an ordained clergyperson. Depending on the denomination, baptism may entail anything from a sprinkle of water on the head to total immersion in water. The age at which one is baptized also varies; some denominations teach that infants should be baptized at birth, while others believe that baptism should be held off until a person is old enough to choose the faith for him or herself.

Denominations that baptize *infants* include:

- Anglican;
- Eastern Orthodox;
- Lutheran;
- Methodist; and
- Roman Catholic.

The Presbyterian Church and the United Church of Christ sometimes baptize infants to indicate membership into the church family, although this is sometimes postponed until the individual can make the choice of membership for him or herself.

Denominations that follow *adult baptism*, typically with full immersion in water, include:

- Baptist;
- Church of Christ; and
- Pentecostal.

Significant exceptions include Quakers, who do not carry out baptism as a religious practice, believing instead in an inward purification of the spirit, and Mormons, who are traditionally baptized at age eight.

Although baptism is not typically performed in the hospital, there are two important times when it may become an issue. First, a Christian patient who was not baptized at birth may wish to be baptized if death is imminent. Second, Christian parents may wish to have a baby baptized if the child is very ill because they fear that the baby will not go to heaven if s/he is not baptized; this can be a cause of great distress for parents.

Holy Communion (also called the Eucharist) is also a key ritual for many Christians and involves consuming bread and wine (or juice) that has been blessed and distributed by clergy. This is a re-creation of Jesus' final meal with his followers. During that meal, called the Last Supper, Jesus offered his closest disciples bread and wine to symbolize his body and blood (some Christians believe the bread and wine are representations of Jesus' body and blood, while others believe them to be Jesus' literal body and blood). Communion may be taken on Sundays, holidays, or at any time that clergy deem it to be appropriate, though it usually occurs during worship services.

Many congregations have clergy or lay people who visit hospitals and administer Communion for patients unable to attend a traditional worship service. Preparations for taking Communion vary among different Christian traditions. Some denominations, particularly Roman Catholicism, teach that one must fast for at least 1 hour (and make confession—see below) prior to receiving Communion. A Catholic patient may wish to have his/her mealtimes or medication schedule adjusted so that the fasting can take place prior to Communion.

Confession prior to taking Communion is another practice followed by some denominations. Both Eastern Orthodox Christians and Roman Catholics may wish to confess to a priest either before receiving Communion or when seriously ill. Roman Catholicism teaches that priests have been given divine authority to forgive the sins committed by believers. In order to be absolved of sins, and thus to restore one's connection to God's grace, believers must confess their sins to a priest. The priest then prays for the penitent, who in turn makes a prayer acknowledging his/her faults before God.

Confession is less formal in the Eastern Orthodox tradition. Generally, Orthodox Christians choose a trusted spiritual guide to whom they make confession; this is often a parish priest, but can be anyone that has received permission from the bishop to hear confessions.

Sunday is the traditional day of worship for the majority of Christian denominations (some observe the Sabbath on Saturday, notably Seventh-day Adventists). On this day, many Christians attend church, where they worship with their faith community through prayer, hymns, readings from the Bible, and messages from clergy. If patients are unable to attend a formal service, they may receive visits from family and/or spiritual leaders, who will likely pray with them, and possibly read from the Bible or offer Communion. Some may wish to view televised services if available.

Most Christians will not object to receiving treatments or having procedures performed on Sundays, although some may prefer to have them done on other days if possible. A notable exception is Seventh-day Adventists, who may refuse treatment on Friday evenings and Saturdays as part of their Sabbath observance.

Jehovah's Witnesses do not observe a Sabbath, believing that every day is holy. Instead, they gather for five meetings each week:

- A Public Talk by an elder, usually on Sundays;

- A lesson based on an article from the *Watchtower*, the Jehovah's Witness official publication, often directly following the Public Talk;

- Theocratic Ministry School, training in how to engage in ministry more effectively;

- A Service Meeting, training on preaching and teaching, usually after Theocratic Ministry School; and

- Book Study, when believers gather to study the latest issue of the *Watchtower*.

Patients who are unable to attend these sessions may be visited by family, co-congregants, or elders for prayer or *Watchtower* study.

Practitioners working with Christian patients from Eastern Orthodox traditions may come into contact with icons, which are extremely important in Orthodox religious practice. Icons are images painted onto flat panels; the subject is traditionally a divine being or subject like Jesus Christ or an angel. Icons adorn most Orthodox Christian churches, and many Orthodox Christian believers have a special place in their homes to hang icons.

Accordingly, many will choose to bring their icons with them to the hospital. Icons are not objects of worship, but rather provide the worshiper with a material symbol that reminds him/her of the presence of the divine. Patient permission is necessary before touching the objects, which should be handled carefully.

Additionally, patients from all Christian denominations may wish to read the Bible and/or pray, either individually or with other Christians. Christians believe that praying and reading the Bible provide spiritual strength, especially during times of illness. A quiet space to pray for those mobile enough would be appreciated.

HYGIENE & WASHING REQUIREMENTS

Generally, there are no hygiene or washing requirements for Christian patients.

DIETARY REQUIREMENTS

There are no overarching dietary rules in Christianity, but many denominations have their own particular regulations.

Roman Catholics may wish to fast before receiving Communion and abstain from eating meat on Fridays; this is more likely to be observed during Lent, the 40 days preceding Easter (Easter, which is the most important holiday in the Christian calendar, commemorates Jesus Christ's death and resurrection and typically occurs anywhere from late March to late April). During Lent, many Christians prepare for Easter by attending extra worship services, and there is a greater emphasis on prayer, penitence, almsgiving, and self-denial.

Strict Orthodox Christians observe a number of fasting times throughout the year, including fasting on Wednesdays and Fridays, and abstaining from meat and dairy products; those with health problems are not expected to observe the fast, though some may still wish to do so.

Mormons often fast on the first Sunday of each month, and typically abstain from consuming anything containing alcohol, coffee, or tea. Some, but not all, Mormons see this as a prohibition on caffeine and will not, for example, drink caffeinated cola drinks. These prohibitions in the Mormon tradition are found in their health code, known as the *Word of Wisdom*.

For Seventh-day Adventists, most of whom also abstain from alcohol and caffeine, abstention is based on the teaching of "healthful living," which emphasizes the importance of making decisions that give the believer an advantage in the development of his/her body, mind, and soul. Many Seventh-day Adventists also interpret this principle as requiring a vegetarian diet.

The Jehovah's Witness tradition teaches that blood should not be ingested because it has special meaning to God, and that violation of this rule can lead to a complete dissolution of one's relationship with God. This restriction motivates the commonly known Jehovah's Witness prohibition on blood transfusions, and many Jehovah's Witnesses also interpret it as requiring a vegetarian diet; in particular, the religion warns against eating meat from an animal that has been strangled or shot and not bled properly.

MEDICATION, TREATMENT, OR PROCEDURE RESTRICTIONS

There are variations among some Christian religious denominations on the medication, treatment, and/or procedures they are willing to use.

As noted, Jehovah's Witnesses customarily refuse blood transfusions for both themselves and their children, even in life-threatening situations, due to a teaching that a human must not sustain his/her life with another creature's blood. For Jehovah's Witnesses, the Bible's reference to blood as the "soul of the flesh" means that it is particularly special to God and its consumption is strictly forbidden. Flouting the prohibition may result in excommunication from the faith community.

Consequently, Jehovah's Witnesses typically refuse medical treatment that requires the use or transfusion of blood or blood products, which includes whole blood, red cells, white cells, platelets, and plasma. Some Jehovah's Witnesses allow auto-transfusion (where the patient's own blood is collected and re-infused) as long as the blood is not stored and is returned immediately to the patient via continuous circuit. Blood samples may be taken for testing, provided any unused blood is disposed of, and non-blood substances (e.g., replacement fluids and blood substitutes) may be infused into the bloodstream.

Although the prohibition on blood products is absolute, there may be differences among some Witnesses on blood-related compounds like albumin and immunoglobulins. There is no rule governing these components, and each individual Witness is free to decide for him or herself whether s/he will accept them.

Many Seventh-day Adventists will refuse medications that contain alcohol or animal byproducts due to their instruction on "healthful living"; Seventh-day Adventism teaches that the body is a temple and should not be contaminated. Alternate treatments should be sought if this becomes an issue.

Christian Scientists are likely to refuse all pain medication, choosing instead to heal themselves through religious practice. Christian Scientists believe that health is simply an illusion; in order to heal oneself, the mind must triumph over matter. Good health occurs when the mind achieves awareness of itself, which is synonymous with awareness of God. Thus, Christian Science healing is not aimed at removing physical suffering, but at leading the ill person to transform his/her consciousness so that s/he may know God. For Christian Science healing practitioners, the chief method of healing is prayer.

Due to their belief in the superiority of Christian Science healing practices, members from that denomination generally forbid Western surgical procedures, amputations, and biopsies. There are some healing tasks such as setting bones or dressing wounds that are seen as purely "mechanical" and any medical practitioner, regardless of religion, will probably be allowed to perform these procedures. However, it is preferable that they are performed by Christian Scientists, and any other practitioners from other religions should not use medication when performing these procedures. There is a directory of Christian Science maintained in the *Christian Science Journal*.

Christians who are opposed to abortion, regardless of denomination, may be extremely reluctant to have any vaccines that are developed from cell lines derived from aborted human fetuses. The health care provider may wish to bring a clergyperson or chaplain into this sensitive discussion.

GENDER & MODESTY
Most Christians will not object to seeing a provider of the opposite sex. However, more conservative Christians will prefer to see someone of the same sex. Each individual patient should be asked for his/her preference.

ORGAN DONATION
Most Christians have no religious objection to the donation or acceptance of organs.

Christian Scientists generally resist all organ, tissue, and body donations due to their general religious objection to medical procedures that address solely physical (versus spiritual) healing; however, each member is free to make his/her own decision.

Jehovah's Witnesses believe that organ, tissue, or body donation is a personal choice. To accommodate their beliefs against blood transfusions, if Jehovah's Witnesses choose to donate, all blood must be removed from the organs and tissues before being transplanted.

INFORMED CONSENT & PATIENT DECISION MAKING

Generally, Christian patients will make decisions individually, although they may choose to consult members of their faith community. Many will find comfort in the counsel of a trusted spiritual leader if the decision involves sensitive issues, such as what efforts should be made to prolong life after a terminal prognosis.

Jehovah's Witness patients will likely want the elders of their faith community to make important health care decisions. Elders are spiritual leaders charged with organizing the congregation's public ministry, providing religious instruction, and conducting spiritual counseling. The Jehovah's Witness tradition is highly hierarchical, and elders are usually very influential in the lives of congregants.

REPRODUCTIVE HEALTH & FAMILY PLANNING

Beliefs on reproductive health and family planning vary greatly according to the secular, liberal, or conservative orientation of a given denomination or congregation.

Almost all denominations of Christianity view pre- and extramarital sex as sinful and teach that sex is only appropriate within the constraints of marriage. Homosexuality is also considered to be sinful by many. Some denominations accept lesbian, gay, bisexual and transsexual members as long as they abstain from sexual activity, while an increasing number accept them without that proscription. Other denominations are reconsidering their positions.

Teachings on family planning vary widely. Some Christians view all forms of family planning as acceptable. Others adamantly oppose all forms of intervention, including artificial contraception, infertility treatment, and voluntary sterilization, believing that God's plan for humanity is for sexual intercourse to be procreative and that contraception disrupts God's natural plan. Most Christian denominations teach abstinence until marriage; discussing premarital sexual relations may cause discomfort for more conservative Christians, or may be problematic for minors.

Although most denominations of Christianity have clear positions on matters of reproductive health and family planning, individual believers are often at odds with the official teachings of their churches. It is critical to discuss a particular patient's beliefs with him/her.

Most Christian denominations are also opposed to abortion, believing that life begins at conception; this means that abortion is equivalent to infanticide. Denominations that have officially announced their opposition to abortion include:

- Roman Catholic (also officially opposed to contraception);
- Eastern Orthodox Christian;
- Episcopalian; and
- Anglican.

In other traditions, abortion is strongly discouraged but is accepted as a last-resort option or when the woman's life is threatened; these include:

- Lutheran;
- Methodist; and
- Presbyterian.

Christians with strong antiabortion sentiments may also be reluctant to have prenatal testing. Again, it is important to remember that there is wide variety among believers' attitudes, and it is important that providers allow patients to express their personal beliefs and preferences.

PREGNANCY & BIRTH

While most Christian traditions readily access medical care in connection with pregnancy and birth, some denominations may require special consideration.

Because blood transfusions are strictly prohibited for Jehovah's Witnesses, extra care should be taken with women during labor and with their infants to ensure that the infants do not become anemic. If providers must draw blood from the baby, a minimum amount should be taken and any extra blood from the sample should be disposed and not used for testing.

Some Christian Scientists prefer to have their children at home, aided by midwives. Those who go to a hospital to give birth will likely wish to minimize the use of medication during labor; most will also wish to return home the same day as the delivery. However, if it is medically necessary for the infant to remain in the hospital, many Christian Scientists will consent.

Different traditions have differing beliefs surrounding the meaning of baptism. Only some denominations have the practice of baptizing at birth, so it is important to discuss baptismal preferences with parents. Denominations that baptize infants include Anglicans, Eastern Orthodox, Lutheran, Methodist, and Roman Catholic; additionally, the Presbyterian Church and the United Church of Christ sometimes baptize infants.

Most denominations that baptize at birth have a formal ceremony in the first few months of the child's life; this is typically done in a church. If a child must be baptized in the hospital, a private room should be provided for the family.

If the birth is very premature or if the infant is seriously ill, some Christians may wish to have their babies baptized by clergy shortly after the birth, believing that this is necessary for the baby's well-being in the afterlife. In many denominations, baptism is considered necessary for salvation:

- Jehovah's Witness;
- Pentecostal;
- Revivalist;
- Roman Catholic; and
- Seventh-day Adventist.

In contrast, most Orthodox and Protestant denominations teach that baptism is only a symbolic ritual or outward sign of one's membership into the Christian community with no implications for one's eternal salvation. Members of these traditions may be less likely to request infant baptism if the infant is ill.

There is no official religious ceremony that is performed universally for Christian miscarriages. Some Christians will want to have their baby blessed and/or baptized by clergy, while some will follow denominational teaching that baptism is a sacrament only for the living. The parents may also wish to have a naming service.

END OF LIFE

For most Christians, death marks the end only of the physical body. All denominations teach that believers' spirits will experience some form of eternal life.

Most Christians will want to be visited by clergy and family prior to death. Visitors will likely pray with the observant patient and/or read from the Bible. Some Christians who have not been previously baptized may wish to have this ritual performed. In emergency situations when a clergyperson or chaplain is not available, baptisms may be performed by a layperson who the patient trusts. Others may wish to receive Communion, depending on their denomination.

Some denominations reject palliative care that would have the side-effect of shortening the patient's life. However, some churches, like the Episcopal and Lutheran churches, have voiced a commitment to the "prevention of intolerable suffering," and allow pain relief that might not defer death.

Roman Catholicism has a special sacrament for the end of life, called *Extreme Unction*, more commonly called *Last Rites*. The Last Rites for Roman Catholics include anointing of the sick, penance (confession), and the Eucharist. First, the dying person is asked, if physically able, to confess. Then, a priest anoints the person on the forehead with oil, usually in the shape of a cross; this is followed by anointing of the hands. Finally, the patient is given communion; bread and wine given to a dying person are called the *viaticum*, meaning "provisions for a journey."

Direct euthanasia is forbidden by most Christian denominations. Patients may seek counsel from a trusted spiritual leader if there is a question of how long life should be prolonged. This is often a question of what God's will is for the patient (i.e., whether it is God's will to prolong human life given its inherent value or to let nature take its course). Chaplains may be a useful resource for the patient when making these difficult decisions.

Christian Scientists are likely to resist medical treatment, even in life-threatening situations. Similarly, Jehovah's Witnesses will likely refuse blood transfusions and blood products for both themselves and their children regardless of the prognosis, because of the teaching that voluntarily accepting it will exclude them from heaven.

Most Christians will be comfortable with a ward's normal practice for handling bodies after death. However, Christian Scientists prefer if female bodies are handled and prepared for burial by women.

There are no formal religious objections to postmortems for many Christian denominations. However, some Christians believe that the body must be intact in order for proper resurrection. A notable example of those who discourage autopsies is Orthodox Christianity. If one is necessary for an Orthodox Christian, every effort should be made to return all the organs to the body, as the body must remain intact for Orthodox burial rites.

FOR MORE READING: CHRISTIANITY

Bellamy, P. Christianity and Medicine. In: Goodacre D, ed. *World Religions and Medicine*. 2nd ed. Oxford, UK: Institute of Religion and Medicine. 1983: 62-71.

Ethnicity Online (2003). Cultural Awareness in Healthcare: Catholics. Ethnicity Online web site http://www.ethnicityonline.net/christianity_catholics.htm. Accessed November 12, 2008.

Ethnicity Online (2003). Cultural Awareness in Healthcare: Christian Scientists. Ethnicity Online web site http://www.ethnicityonline.net/christian_scientists.htm. Accessed November 12, 2008.

Ethnicity Online (2003). Cultural Awareness in Healthcare: Jehovah's Witnesses. Ethnicity Online web site http://www.ethnicityonline.net/jehovahs_witnesses.htm. Accessed November 12, 2008.

Schott J, Henley A. Christianity. In: Schott J, Henley A, eds. *Culture, Religion and Childbearing in a Multiracial Society*. Oxford, UK: Butterworth-Heinemann. 1996: 288-301.

Schott J, Henley A. Jehovah's Witnesses. In: Schott J, Henley A, eds. *Culture, Religion and Childbearing in a Multiracial Society*. Oxford, UK: Butterworth-Heinemann. 1996: 325-28.

3. Islam

Overview FAQ

1. When, where, and how did Islam originate?

In the early seventh century, Muhammad founded Islam in what is now present-day Saudi Arabia, in the city of Mecca (nb: many Muslims, when referring to Muhammad, will add "Peace be upon him" after each mention of his name). A religious, political, and military Arab leader, Muhammad is viewed by Muslims as the last and the greatest of the Prophets sent by the one God (called *Allah*, the standard word for "God" in Arabic).

Islam is one of the three Abrahamic religious traditions (the others are Judaism and Christianity). Thus, Muslims do not believe that Muhammad created the religion itself, but rather that he restored the faith in the one true God proclaimed by Prophets throughout history.

Adherents of Islam are called Muslims.

2. Does Islam have sacred texts? What are they called?

The central text of Islam is the *Qur'an*, which Muslims believe to be the literal word of Allah. Muslims believe that the text of the Qur'an was revealed word for word to Muhammad by the angel Gabriel in the seventh century. The Qur'an is divided into 114 chapters (called *suras*), which lay out core Muslim beliefs, practices, and laws.

The words and deeds of Muhammad during his life were also recorded by his contemporaries and are collected in a set of scriptures called the *Hadith*. The Hadith are regarded as further important guidelines for the Muslim way of life and address some questions not addressed in the Qur'an.

3. What are the core beliefs of Islam?

There are six core beliefs that the majority of Muslims share, called the *Aqidah* ("creed" in Arabic). The first and most fundamental concept is belief in the oneness of God (Allah in Arabic). The Prophet Muhammad is believed to be Allah's last messenger. The other five major beliefs are:

- **Belief in all God's messengers**, which includes belief in Muhammad, Jesus, Moses, and Abraham, among others, as divinely inspired teachers;

- **Belief in God's holy scriptures**, as revealed to the messengers (i.e., the Hebrew Bible/Old Testament, New Testament, and Qur'an);

- **Belief in a final day of judgment** when all people, both Muslim and non-Muslim, will be held accountable for their actions and judged by Allah;

- **Belief in angels**, who are responsible for the laws and workings of nature; and

- **Belief in fate** (i.e., God's divine plan for the world).

4. What are the core practices of Islam?

Individual Muslims may practice their faith in a variety of ways, but there are five major practices recognized by all Muslims, known as the *Five Pillars of Islam:*

- **Shahadah**, or "declaration of faith." To be a Muslim, one must declare the belief that there is only one God, and that Muhammad is his final prophet.

- **Salat**, or "prayers." Muslims are required to pray five times a day, facing in the direction of Mecca and the *Ka'bah*, a building in Mecca believed to have been built by Abraham. Prayers are recited in Arabic and may be performed anywhere, although a *mosque* (Muslim house of worship) is preferable. It is customary for Muslims to ritually cleanse themselves before praying; this often involves washing the face, hands, and feet, although precise practice varies. Prayers typically last between 5 and 15 minutes.

    In addition to the daily prayers, many Muslims also attend a congregational prayer midday on Friday, in which they hear a special sermon given by an *imam* (an Islamic leader, often the leader of a mosque).

- **Sawm**, or "fasting." Muslims are required to abstain from both food and water from dawn to sunset in the month of Ramadan. Islam follows a lunar calendar, and the lunar year is 11 days shorter than the solar year. Thus, while Ramadan always falls during the ninth month in the Islamic lunar calendar, it rotates through the different solar months.

- **Zakat**, or "alms." Muslims are required to give alms to the poor in the amount of 2.5% of excess wealth annually.

- **Hajj**, or "pilgrimage." Muslims are required to make a pilgrimage to Mecca (in Saudi Arabia) once in a lifetime, if they are physically and financially capable of doing so. The hajj begins two months after Ramadan and includes rituals that commemorate the lives of Abraham, patriarch of Muslims, his concubine Hagar, and their son Ishmael.

5. What are Islam's important holidays? How are they celebrated?

Ramadan is the ninth and holiest month of the Islamic year, and is meant to be a time of spiritual and physical purification commemorating the revelation of the Qur'an to Muhammad. Prayers, fasting, charity, and self-accountability are stressed throughout Ramadan, and there are several important days that occur within the month, including *Laylat al-Qadr* and *Eid al-Fitr*.

Laylat al-Qadr commemorates the night that the Qur'an's first verse was revealed to Muhammad. Since the exact night is not known, Muslims often hold prayer vigils throughout the last ten days of Ramadan.

Eid al-Fitr is "The Festival of Breaking the Fast" and marks the end of Ramadan. It begins after sunset on the last day of Ramadan and traditionally lasts for three days. It is customary for food to be donated to the poor, for people to wear their best clothes, and for prayers to be held in the early morning followed by feasting and visiting friends and relatives.

Another important religious festival for Muslims is *Eid al-Adha*, a four-day celebration that commemorates Abraham's willingness to sacrifice his son Ishmael for Allah. During this time, it is common for special foods to be prepared and for children to receive gifts.

6. How many adherents of Islam (i.e., Muslims) are there in the United States? Are they located in a particular region?

Though the statistics concerning the presence of Muslims in the United States are not as comprehensive as would be ideal, there is a general consensus that there are approximately 5 million Muslims in the United States. Some estimates go as high as 7 million. Muslim populations are most concentrated in the Washington-Boston Corridor, Houston, Michigan, and Southern California.

7. What are the main sects or denominations within Islam?

There are two major denominations of Muslims: *Sunni* and *Shi'a*. Though their core beliefs are the same, there are significant differences involving religious leadership and certain applications of Islamic law.

The core difference between Sunni and Shi'a Muslims is that Shi'a believe that the leader of Muslims can only be someone descended directly from the Prophet Muhammad, while the Sunni believe that the most qualified person in the community should rule.

Sunni Muslims form the largest denomination of Islam. Their attitude toward leadership stems from their belief that Muhammad died without naming a successor. According to Sunni teachings, the first *caliph* (head of the Islamic community) after Muhammad's death was chosen based on his capabilities, not his lineage. Accordingly, Sunni do not believe that there is a hereditary class of spiritual leaders. Rather, they believe that leadership of the community is a trust that must be earned and that the Qu'ran and Hadith are the only sources of Islamic rule.

Shi'a Muslims are the second largest denomination of Islam and they believe that Muhammad ordered that all Muslim imams (religious leaders) come from his own bloodline. Shi'as regard the descendants of Muhammad as being infallible and sinless, and treat their authority with special respect.

Sufism is a much smaller tradition within Islam. Believers strive to obtain a direct experience of God through practices including meditation and dance. Some identify Sufism as the mystical practice of Islam. Sufism is not necessarily exclusive of other Muslim denominations; many Sufi orders are associated with Sunni or Shi'a sects.

• • • •

Intersections with Health Care: FAQ

1. Does Islam have a particular view about what causes illness? Are there illness-related rituals?

Most Muslims believe that the fate of their health is determined by Allah.

Some Muslims believe that illness and health-related pain is: 1) sent to them by Allah as a test of faith; 2) bestowed on them by Allah; or 3) a result of not following the Qur'an. Observant/traditional Muslims, including those from an older generation, may view their illness as something that is to be endured and from which they are expected to learn. However, most Muslims have a great deal of respect for the field of medicine and Islam teaches that it is the responsibility of the individual to maintain the body given to them by Allah.

2. Does Islam prescribe a particular type of dress for men and/or women?

Many Muslims, especially women, have strict beliefs surrounding modesty and the importance of modest attire; many believe that Islam requires women to cover their hair, torso, legs, and arms while in public. Consequently, Muslim women may choose to wear modest clothes, ranging from a simple head scarf to full-body robes. Muslim men may also choose to wear a head covering, often a brimless cap. For men, it is also important that the area between the waist and knees not be exposed.

Some Muslim women may also wear jewelry that has religious significance, such as a marriage bangle. Both genders may wear charms that have excerpts from the Qur'an written on them; the charms are often given by family members to promote health. These also should not be removed without consent whenever possible.

If a Muslim patient needs to be examined, they may wish to expose only the relevant part of the body, while keeping the rest of the body covered. If possible, the patient should be provided with modest clothing (covering the ankles, arms, and throat, and with a closed back).

Some Muslim men may choose to grow facial hair as a way of following the tradition begun by Muhammad. Providers may face resistance when a particular procedure requires shaving. Where possible, alternatives should be pursued.

3. Are there any prayer or ritual observances that are likely to occur during the Muslim patient's stay?

Devout Muslims pray five times a day (called salat). The precise cleansing practices used by an individual patient vary (see the Q & A below on cleansing). Customarily, Muslims ritually cleanse themselves with running water before each prayer. Additionally, if their clothing is unclean, a patient may wish to change before prayer. Most Muslims use a prayer mat to sit, kneel, stand, or lie on during prayers. Ideally, prayers are conducted in an undisturbed, quiet space. Patients may request that hospital staff wake them up at certain times so that they can prepare for prayer.

Islam provides some health-based exceptions from prayer, including: women who have given birth less than 40 days ago; women who are menstruating; men or women suffering from mental health problems; and the seriously ill. Notwithstanding these "exceptions," Muslim patients who fall into the last two categories may still want to pray.

There is congregational prayer every Friday required of Muslim men. Customarily, men attend a service in a mosque, where they hear readings and messages from an imam. Attendance is optional for women, who are seated in a separate section of the mosque. If, for health reasons, a Muslim patient is unable to attend the Friday prayer, an imam or Muslim religious leader may visit. To the extent possible, try to allow privacy for these visits.

4. Does Islam have hygiene or washing requirements?

Many Muslims ritually cleanse themselves before prayer. Rituals include prescribed movements, such as washing the face from brow to chin, rinsing the hands from wrist to fingertips, and cleansing the nostrils, mouth, and ears three times. For those unable to access running water, a symbolic sequence of gestures for the cleansing may be performed. Some observant Muslims may also request a jug of water and a bowl.

5. Are there any dietary restrictions?

Islam teaches that there are certain foods that were declared by Allah as permissible, or *halal*. Whether meat is halal depends on the way the animal was killed and treated after death. Islam also teaches that pork or anything containing pork products is strictly prohibited, regardless of how the animal was killed. Some Muslims also consider fish without fins or scales to be *haram*, or forbidden.

In addition to non-halal meat, Muslims traditionally do not consume anything that contains alcohol, any animal blood or blood products, or fish without fins or scales.

Given their adherence to a halal diet, Muslim patients may be hesitant to consume anything in a health care facility, fearing cross-contamination between halal and non-halal food. If possible, provide either certifiably halal food or a vegetarian alternative. Because the rules for kosher food are similar, many Muslims will eat certifiably kosher food, but this needs to be checked with the patient.

During Ramadan, Islam requires that Muslims 12 years of age or older undergo a month-long fast. During this period, Muslims do not consume food or liquid between sunrise and sunset. Meals are allowed after a prayer at sunset and before sunrise. Those whose health would be compromised by fasting are permitted to disregard this practice, though many still follow it.

6. Are there any medications, treatments, or procedures that adherents of Islam (i.e., Muslims) cannot accept?

Some patients may be reluctant to take pain medication, believing that the pain is a test of their faith. However, Islam teaches that it is allowable to take medication that alleviates pain if it is not narcotic or intoxicating.

A common issue that arises is resistance to taking medicine during Ramadan. Those healthy enough to observe Ramadan may oppose injections, liquid and solid medication, intravenous drips, and even nasal sprays, because fasting prohibits the intake of anything through an open route into the body. If any of these is necessary for the health of the patient, the health care provider may want to speak with both the imam and the patient. Often, the fast can be accommodated by adjusting the timing of medication or using skin patches, or topical or sublingual medications.

7. Can Muslim patients who follow Islamic tradition see providers of the opposite sex?

A traditional tenet of Islam is that men and women should be segregated in public. Any physical contact (e.g., handshakes) between people of opposite genders is discouraged, as it is regarded as a dangerous temptation to improper sexual contact. Thus, providers should approach Muslims of the opposite gender with extreme sensitivity. If possible, offer providers of the same sex. If this is not possible, women may request a female to be present, while married females may be accompanied by their husbands.

8. Can Muslim patients who follow Islamic tradition donate organs or accept donor organs?

As a general rule, Muslims will only allow organ donation if both the donor and recipient are Muslim; organs should not be taken for storage. Additionally, transplantation is admissible only if necessary for the recipient's life.

9. Should I consult anyone in addition to the patient himself/herself when seeking informed consent or other patient decisions?

Traditionally, Muslim men are considered the protectors of their wives and children. Muslim women who uphold this belief may refuse treatment without a husband's or father's consent.

10. What are Islam's views on reproductive health and family planning? Are contraceptives accepted? What about abortion? Voluntary sterilization?

In general, married Muslims are allowed to use contraceptive methods that prevent conception (e.g., a condom or birth control pill) but *not* contraceptives that would prevent a fertilized ovum from being successfully implanted; this is considered akin to abortion. Birth control pills and the rhythm method are common among observant Muslims. For very observant Muslims, contraception is only permissible if it is used to avoid a pregnancy that would harm either the woman or the fetus. However, some observant Muslims discourage all forms of family planning, believing that Allah decides when to bestow the blessing of children.

In vitro fertilization is normally permissible only if every other form of conception has been ruled out. Donated eggs or sperm are not acceptable. Collecting sperm for infertility testing or in vitro treatments may also be problematic among highly observant Muslims, many of whom consider masturbation to be sinful. Collecting semen for the purpose of diagnosis or therapy, however, is permissible.

Islam teaches that at four months, angels breathe life into the flesh of the fetus. Thus, termination of the pregnancy after this period is considered infanticide. The only admissible exception is when the mother's life is in danger.

Generally, voluntary sterilization is discouraged. Hysterectomies are to be used only as a last resort. Muslim husbands often prefer to be present whenever reproductive health or sterilization is discussed.

11. Are there particular beliefs or rituals concerning pregnancy and birth? What about postpartum women? What about women who have miscarried?

Immediately after birth, it is traditional for Muslim babies to be washed. Some Muslims believe that the first sound the baby should hear is the whispering of a call to prayer into the right and then the left ear by the child's father or a male relative.

Some Muslims may wish to shave the newborn's head between three and seven days postbirth to remove the impurities of birth; this ceremony is called the *aqiqah*; this is a pre-Islamic Arab tradition that some Muslims believe is religious and culturally mandated. The hair itself is often buried. On the day of the aqiqah, infants receive their proper name. In conjunction with the naming ceremony, parents may also wish to circumcise a newborn boy.

Traditionally, Muslim women do not leave their house for 40 days after birth. If the new mother needs medical attention, she may prefer to have a home visit. Muslim mothers will most likely wish to breastfeed.

If miscarriage occurs after the fourth month of pregnancy, parents may wish to name the child and give him/her a traditional burial. Health care providers touching the fetus should wear gloves and wrap the birth products in a clean, white cloth. If possible, the placenta and any other birth products should also be given to the family for burial.

12. Are there end-of-life rituals or beliefs I need to know about?

For many Muslims, death is accepted as a normal and necessary step between life in the material world and life with Allah. Although Muslims believe that Allah plans the correct time of death, medical support should be given for as long as possible.

Patients and their families may be distressed by the idea of a DNR, thinking it implies that everything is not being done to sustain life. If such a case arises, an imam may help mediate the conversation. Additionally, Islam teaches that there is a condition called "movement of the slain" when a person may be termed dead despite movement, such as when a patient is brain-dead but breathing with the aid of a ventilator. In these cases, the family and an imam should be consulted for next steps, if at all possible.

Muslim patients may wish to die at home in the care of their family and friends. If this is not possible, most Muslims will wish to be surrounded by loved ones, and hospitals should anticipate a large number of visitors. Since visitors may wish to help care for the sick, the provider may need to articulate what care is best for the patient.

As death approaches, prayers and passages from the Qur'an are recited. Additionally, the patient may wish for their bed to be positioned so that their head faces Mecca. If possible, the last words a Muslim says will be the shahadah, a declaration of faith.

13. What should be done with the body after death?

Islam teaches that the soul of the deceased is freed from the body upon death. Muslims believe that the body is resurrected after death, so it must be handled carefully.

If possible, providers should wear gloves, turn the patient's head toward Mecca, straighten the legs and arms, and close the mouth and eyes. The body should be covered with a clean, white cloth. Providers should not wash the body, but when possible, should reserve this task for a family member of the same sex who cleanses the body with scented water. Female bodies are traditionally dressed in five robes and males in three, over which a shroud is placed.

The family may wish to pray in privacy before the body is taken to the morgue. Typically, the family will request that the body be released as quickly as possible so that it can be prepared for burial.

Most Muslim families will not allow a postmortem to be performed, as it is considered desecration of the body and is thus forbidden (haram). If a postmortem is absolutely necessary, great care should be taken to return all of the organs to the body and close all wounds.

• • • •

Islam: Intersections with Health Care

The word Islam is Arabic and means "peace through submission to God." Muslims are the people who follow the religion of Islam; Muslims accept that their lives will be spent in submission to the will of God (or Allah) and in obedience to the teachings of Muhammad, his prophet (n.b.: many Muslims, when referring to Muhammad, will add "Peace be upon him" after each mention of his name).

A key manner in which Muslims practice submission to Allah is by assuming responsibility for respecting the body Allah has provided. This includes the duty to seek medical treatment when necessary, even though one's fate is ultimately determined by Allah. The Islamic world was one of the first to take a scientific approach to the practice of medicine and the observation of illness. Many of the world's first physicians came from the Islamic community or studied in the Middle East. In Islam, treating another human being in his/her hour of need is viewed as one of the most honorable things a person can do. This is explicitly mentioned in the Qur'an: "That whosoever saves a human life, it is as if they have saved the whole of humankind" (Qur'an, sura 5:32).

Quick answers for many questions that arise when caring for a Muslim patient may be found in the FAQ. For more in-depth explanations, consult the appropriate section below.

CAUSE OF ILLNESS AND HEALING RITUALS

Many observant Muslims see illness and health-related pain as springing from one of three related sources:

1. A trial sent by Allah as a test of faith;

2. Something bestowed by Allah; or

3. The result of not following the directives of the Qur'an, including proper care of one's body.

Orthodox Muslims or those from older generations may view their illnesses as things to be endured and from which they must learn. Islamic texts have many examples of Muhammad's followers embracing their injuries and illnesses as opportunities to demonstrate the strength of their faith and to deepen their connections to Allah.

Despite these beliefs, most Muslims have great respect for the field of medicine and for medical practitioners. Health care providers are seen as conduits through which Allah directs his will. In addition, because Islam teaches that it is the responsibility of the individual to take care of the body Allah has given to them, medical treatment is to be obtained when needed.

DRESS & MODESTY

The nature of Islamic modesty requirements is currently a topic of much debate within and outside the Muslim community. Some vehemently maintain that extensive coverage of both hair and body is required by the Qur'an. Other Muslims disagree that it is an undisputed religious duty, seeing questions of how to dress modestly as matters of personal choice that are subject to individual and cultural interpretation.

Regardless, many Muslims, women and men alike, have strict beliefs surrounding modesty in clothing. For women in particular, Islam teaches that modest dress is important because it allows the woman to be appreciated for attributes other than the physical.

Thus, observant Muslims generally agree that women have a duty to keep their hair covered, and many Muslim women choose to wear modest clothing and/or some form of head or full-body covering. Common garments include:

- The *hijab*, a scarf usually worn wrapped around the head, neck, and shoulders. Depending on how the individual woman chooses to wear the hijab, more or less of her face may remain visible. This may be worn with one of the other traditional garments or with Western-style clothing.

- The *niqab*, a head covering that leaves only the eyes visible.

- The *jilbab*, a long, loose coat that covers the entire body except the hands, feet, and face. It is typically worn together with hijab or niqab.

- The *burkha*, a cloak-like garment that covers the entire body from head to feet, worn over and in addition to a woman's clothing.

Due to their religious significance, these garments should not be removed without patient consent. If they must be removed before consent can be obtained, providers should place the garments in a clean, safe location and may want to offer a surgical cap or face mask so the patient can maintain some coverage. Some Muslim women will also feel uncomfortable in typical hospital garments. If options are available, they should be offered a long garment with a high neckline that does not gape in the back. If there are no acceptable options, women may wish to wear a shawl over their hospital robes.

Some Muslim women may also wear jewelry that has religious significance, such as a marriage bangle, and both genders may wear charms that have excerpts from the Qur'an written on them; the charms are often given by family members to promote health. As with modest garments, they should not be removed without consent, and should be treated respectfully if they must be removed.

Muslim men are also exhorted to dress modestly; for them, modesty requirements dictate that the body be covered from navel to knees. Typically, Western dress meets these requirements, so it is less common in the United States to see Muslim men in traditional dress. Many men do wear a head covering, usually a small, brimless cap. This cap should be treated in the same way as women's garments.

In addition, some Muslim men may choose to grow out their facial hair in emulation of the Prophet Muhammad. Therefore, the health care provider may face resistance when a procedure requires the shaving of the face; this should be discussed with the patient in advance.

GENDER & MODESTY

Some Muslims do not allow physical contact with an individual of the opposite sex, whether the individual is a Muslim or non-Muslim, due to traditional tenets on gender segregation in public. Thus, health care providers should approach Muslims of the opposite gender with extreme sensitivity. If possible, health care providers of the same sex as the patient should be offered. If this is not possible, women and girls may request that a female be present or bring a chaperone; married females may be accompanied by their husbands. Men may also prefer same-sex caregivers.

This concern for gender segregation may also extend to the hospital ward in which a patient is housed; more observant Muslims may be averse to being in gender-mixed wards.

Even with practitioners of the same sex, some Muslims may remain hesitant to discuss sexual activity. It is generally considered a very private matter that is kept confidential between a husband and wife. Speaking about sexual preferences and practices is more than just a taboo; it is considered haram or "unclean." While it may be allowable in the context of treatment, great sensitivity must be shown by the practitioner to meet both the health *and* religious needs of the patient.

Regardless of the respective gender of the patient and health care practitioner, Muslim patients may be reluctant to expose their legs, chests, or genitals. The patient will likely only expose the area of his/her body that needs medical attention.

PRAYER & RITUAL OBSERVANCES

Devout Muslims pray five times a day (this requirement is called salat). The times of daily prayer follow the position of the sun and occur:

1. At dawn;

2. When the sun is at its apex;

3. At the time in the afternoon when the sun casts a shadow equal in length to the height of a person;

4. At sunset; and

5. In total darkness.

Prayer times, therefore, vary with the seasons. In addition, some Shi'a Muslims may combine prayer times and pray three times a day instead of five; providers should check with their individual patients. Patients may request that hospital staff wake them up at certain times so that they can prepare for prayer. Providers should make an effort to find out when prayer times will occur and avoid scheduling procedures or tests during those periods.

Though it is always preferable to pray in a mosque, prayer can also be observed in an appropriate clean, dry place, which can be created virtually anywhere by placing a prayer rug or other clean covering (such as a towel) on the ground. Patients should be afforded as much privacy as possible during prayer times; hospitalized patients who are not confined to their beds may be more comfortable in a separate room such as a quiet space or in an inclusive hospital chapel.

Traditionally, Islamic prayer is highly physical and involves adherents standing, bowing, and prostrating themselves on the floor. Patients with limited mobility may encounter difficulties performing prayer in their customary ways and may require assistance. However, they are allowed to pray sitting, or while lying in bed. In these situations, it may be advisable to have the patient's imam or a chaplain visit to discuss modifications to the traditional prayer ritual.

Even in preparing for prayer, physical exertion may be needed. Many Muslims ritually cleanse themselves (with ritual ablutions called *wudu*) with running water (see Hygiene & Washing Requirements) to purify the mind and body before beginning prayer. Traditionally, wudu requires washing the face (including the ears, nose, and mouth), hands, and feet. Again, patients with limited mobility may have difficulty accessing a source of running water, requiring either assistance or a jug of water.

If washing with water is difficult or undesirable from a medical point of view, one type of adaptation would involve a Muslim patient performing *tayamum*, or waterless ablution. To perform tayamum, a person touches a natural substance (e.g., a stone) and uses their hands to wipe the face and forearms. A bedridden patient may perform tayamum by first patting a pillow.

If the patient's clothing is unclean, s/he may also wish to change into clean clothes before prayer.

Muslim teachings recognize exceptions from salat obligations when it may jeopardize a person's health. Those exempt include:

- Women who have given birth less than 40 days prior;
- Women who are menstruating;
- Men and women suffering from mental health problems; and
- Men and women who are otherwise seriously ill.

However, Muslim patients who fall into the last two categories may still wish to do their prayers and should certainly be helped to do so if they are physically able.

There is a special communal prayer every Friday required for Muslim men. Customarily, men attend a service in their mosque where they hear readings and messages from the imam and pray together. For Muslim women, attendance is optional, and those who attend are seated in a separate section of the mosque. If, for health reasons, a Muslim patient is unable to attend the Friday prayer, an imam or Muslim religious leader may visit that day. If this happens, health care providers should allow privacy to the extent possible. Alternatively, the patient may listen to audio or television broadcasts or a prayer service, if possible.

HYGIENE & WASHING REQUIREMENTS

As outlined in the section Prayer & Ritual Observance, Muslims ritually cleanse themselves before prayers; this ritual is called *wudu*. This physical cleansing represents the spiritual cleansing of one's mind, body, and soul.

Wudu includes prescribed moves, such as washing the face from brow to chin, rinsing the hands from wrist to fingertips, and cleansing the nostrils, mouth, and ears three times. For those unable to access a source of running water, a symbolic sequence of gestures may be performed without water. However, very observant Muslims may request a jug of water and a bowl.

DIETARY REQUIREMENTS

Islam teaches that there are certain foods that were declared by Allah as permissible (halal), while others were declared impermissible (haram). Eating halal foods is an important religious practice through which Muslims demonstrate discipline that shows their submission to Allah.

Whether meat is halal depends on the type of meat and the way in which the animal was killed. To qualify as halal, the animal must die from a single blow to the throat with a sharp knife while the name of Allah is pronounced over it. Following its death, the animal must be hung up by the hind feet while the blood drains out of its body.

Islam teaches that pork or anything containing pork products is haram, regardless of how the pig was killed. In addition to pork and non-halal meat, Muslims do not consume anything that contains alcohol. Some Muslims also consider fish without fins or scales to be haram, or forbidden.

Given their adherence to a halal diet, Muslim patients may be hesitant to consume anything in the hospital, fearing cross-contamination between halal and non-halal food if the facility does not have a separate halal kitchen with staff who are attuned to Muslim dietary requirements. If possible, the hospital should provide either certifiably halal food from an outside source or a vegetarian alternative; kosher meals may also be acceptable. If hospital policy and the patient's medical status allow, family and friends may also bring halal foods from home; this serves both to guarantee a source of halal food and comfort to the patient.

During Ramadan, Islam teaches that all adherents who have attained puberty should undergo a month-long fast. During this period, Muslims do not consume any food or liquid between dawn and sunset. In fact, they do not ingest anything. Meals are allowed after a prayer at sunset and then until dawn; dates are often used to break the fast at sunset. Staff should be sure that patients consume sufficient water during the night to prepare them for the next fast day.

Those whose health does not allow fasting are excused from this religious practice. This includes people with both temporary and long-term illnesses; these exemptions also include women who are within 40 days of giving birth or those who are menstruating. However, some patients may, nonetheless, be intent on fasting, as they believe that the spiritual benefits of fasting overcome the physiological consequences of refusing food, water, or medicine.

The fast prohibits taking any food or liquid into the body through an open route. This may mean that a Muslim patient may reject all food and even refuse oral and some intravenous medications, injections, and nasal sprays during the fast period of each day of Ramadan; see Medication, Treatment, or Procedure Restrictions.

MEDICATION, TREATMENT, OR PROCEDURE RESTRICTIONS

Some patients may be reluctant to take medication, believing that the pain is a test of their faith. There may also be a reluctance to take medications containing alcohol or other intoxicants, which Islam teaches are forbidden, or haram (see Dietary Requirements). However, Islam teaches that it is allowable to take medication that alleviates pain if it is not intoxicating. Accordingly, if the medication is critical for the patient and the patient is resistant, an imam may be able to help negotiate the decision making by the patient.

Where alternatives exist, medications that contain pork or pork derivatives should be avoided, as should any procedures involving pork products (e.g., a biological heart valve replacement with a porcine valve), because pork is also haram. If there are no non-haram medications or procedures available, the patient may wish to speak with an imam or chaplain before deciding whether to consent to the treatment.

A more common issue that arises is the resistance to taking medicine during Ramadan. Those healthy enough to observe Ramadan will often oppose taking injections, swallowing either liquid or solid medications, intravenous drips, and even nasal sprays, because the fast prohibits the intake of any substance through an open route into the body.

If any of these medications or procedures are necessary for the health of the patient, the health care provider may want to speak with both the patient and an imam. As noted in Dietary Requirements, Islam does provide exemptions to fasting requirements, particularly for the ill. If a patient is adamant, providers can choose to accommodate the fast to the extent possible by adjusting the timing of medications or suggesting the use of a skin patch or topical medication.

INFORMED CONSENT & PATIENT DECISION MAKING

Traditionally, Muslim men are considered the protectors of both their wives and children. For some Muslim women who adhere to this belief, treatment may be refused until a husband's or father's consent is given.

For the most part, this is a cultural practice and is not ordained by Islam. In general, an adult woman can consent for herself. Also, a married woman can consent for herself, except in cases where it affects the husband's gamete (e.g., the use of contraception or sterilization). In most medical situations, there will be no need to obtain a husband's or father's consent.

REPRODUCTIVE HEALTH & FAMILY PLANNING

As discussed in Gender & Modesty, Islam has fairly strict requirements on interaction between the sexes to prevent distractions from Islamic religious requirements; even a handshake may be regarded as temptation. It is not surprising, then, that any sex outside marriage (premarital or extramarital) is haram (i.e., forbidden). When an unmarried Muslim seeks medical attention for an issue related to sexual activity, s/he may, therefore, be uncomfortable and will appreciate extra sensitivity, especially if the patient is a minor or is accompanied by family members who may be unaware of his/her sexual activity.

In general, married Muslims are allowed to use contraceptive methods that prevent conception (e.g., a condom or birth control pill) but *not* contraceptives that would prevent a fertilized ovum from being successfully implanted; this is considered akin to abortion. Birth control pills and the rhythm method are common among observant Muslims. For very observant Muslims, contraception is only permissible if it is used to avoid a pregnancy that would harm either the woman or the fetus.

Some Muslims, married and unmarried, will be highly uncomfortable in physical exams that include a sexual history or physical examination of the sex organs. Every possible effort should be made to provide the patient with a practitioner of the same sex and to allow the patient to bring a family member or chaperone. Teaching hospitals should seek to implement practices that avoid bringing groups of students, especially mixed-gender groups, to these exams.

Questions of infertility should be approached with great care. The woman is traditionally blamed when infertility exists, and the many restrictions around gender and reproductive health may make the procedures for addressing the infertility logistically tricky.

In vitro fertilization is normally permissible, but only when every other form of fertility treatment has been ruled out. The cells used should be the couples' own; donated eggs or sperm are generally not considered acceptable because they call the legitimacy of the child into question (surrogacy is frowned upon for similar reasons). During in vitro fertilization, providers should discuss in advance how any unused embryos will be handled.

Collecting sperm for infertility testing or in vitro treatments may also be problematic among highly observant Muslims, many of whom consider masturbation to be sinful. Collecting semen for the purpose of diagnosis or therapy is permissible. Patients may prefer to collect a sperm sample themselves at home, rather than in a health care facility.

According to Islamic law, termination of a pregnancy is permissible until the fourth month. Islam teaches that at four months, angels breathe life into the flesh of the fetus; thus, termination of the pregnancy after this period is considered infanticide. The only permissible exception is when the mother's life is in danger. Even then, providers must exhaust all other possible treatments before turning to abortion. Notwithstanding Islamic teaching, individuals may have their own strong beliefs on the topic.

Generally, voluntary sterilization for both men and women is discouraged. Thus, hysterectomies are to be a last resort. Providers should note that the woman may face both religious and familial pressure not to undergo the procedure, and should try to make appropriate counseling available. Muslim husbands will often prefer to be present anytime sterilization or reproductive health is discussed with a married Muslim woman.

PREGNANCY & BIRTH

In Islam, children are considered a signal of Allah's favor and are cause for great celebration; they are thought of as a family's wealth.

Immediately after birth, babies should be washed to remove all impurities. Some Muslims believe that the first sound the baby should hear is a whispering call to prayer into its right and left ears by its father or a male relative; it is believed that this helps the newborn understand the duty to Allah from the moment of birth. In the case of a premature infant needing immediate care, parents may wish to do this before the infant is removed to a nursery or NICU.

In some cultures, small pouches may be placed around the neck of Muslim babies soon after birth; this is a cultural practice and is not actually part of Islamic teaching. These pouches contain prayers and words from the Qur'an that are believed to ward off evil. In addition, dates or honey might be placed in the baby's mouth to welcome the child into the sweetness of a good life. Honey, which can contain spores causing infant botulism, is not recommended for newborns; if a family wishes to observe this tradition, work with them to find a non-honey alternative.

In Islam, the placenta is considered to be human flesh. Some parents may not want the hospital or birthing facility to dispose of the placenta, but will wish to bury it. If possible, the placenta should be saved and provided to the parents, if that is their wish.

Some Muslims may wish to shave the newborn's head between three and seven days after birth. This ceremony is called the *aqiqah*; it is a pre-Islamic Arab tradition that some Muslims believe is religiously and culturally mandated.

During the aqiqah, the hair may be weighed and the weight of the hair in silver is given to the poor. The hair itself is often buried. Infants also receive their proper name. Prior to this day, boys are given one of the 99 names of Allah and girls are often called Fatima; infants are not often named at birth. Given the importance of the naming ceremony, an imam may be consulted. The birth certificate and medical records should be updated after this ceremony.

Parents may wish to circumcise a newborn boy. Circumcision (*khitan*) is traditionally done within four weeks of birth, and can be performed before the newborn is discharged from the hospital. Parents may prefer to have this done at home.

Some Muslim women choose not to leave their homes for 40 days after birth to allow them time to rest; this is largely a cultural, not a religious, tenet. If the new mother needs medical attention, she may prefer to have a home visit. Muslim mothers will most likely wish to breastfeed. As the Qur'an states, it is the best way to care for a child, but mothers may be reluctant to discuss the practice with providers.

Some Muslim women who have lost pregnancies may struggle with the concept that the miscarriage was Allah's will or a result of past sins, and may benefit from counseling from a supportive imam or chaplain.

If the pregnancy is lost after the fourth month (when the fetus achieves human form because the soul enters the body), the parents may wish to name the child and give him/her a traditional burial. Any health care provider touching the child should wear gloves and wrap the baby in a clean, white cloth. Washing the body should be left to the family. If possible, the placenta and other non-fetal tissue should also be given to the family for burial.

ORGAN DONATION

Medical advances have led to extensive debate within the Muslim community about how to apply the rules of the Qur'an in modern society. Two common tensions in the debate on organ donation are the religious duty to save a life and the requirement of burying the body intact. The ultimate decision on how to balance this tension is made by the patient and his/her family. However, many Muslims are comfortable with donation.

If the patient or his/her family feels uncomfortable making the decision, an imam or chaplain can be called in to respond to their concerns.

END OF LIFE

For many Muslims, death is accepted as a necessary step between life in the material world and the hereafter. Through this acceptance, Muslims show their total submission to Allah's will. After death, Islam teaches that the soul of the deceased is freed from the body and rejoins friends and family who have already died. It is also believed that although Allah determines each individual's time to die, health care providers are also conduits of Allah's will and medical support should be given for as long as possible.

Patients and their families may be distressed by the idea of making a decision about whether or not to resuscitate. Indeed, a Do Not Resuscitate order may be viewed as implying that everything is not being done to sustain the patient's life. In this case, an imam may help mediate the conversation.

Generally, Muslims accept brain death as the moment of death. Additionally, Islam teaches that there is a condition called "movement of the slain," when a person may be declared dead despite some physical movement; this applies to patients who are brain-dead but breathing with the aid of a ventilator. In this case, the family and an imam should be consulted for next steps.

Muslim patients may wish to die at home in the care of their family and friends. If this is not possible, most hospitalized Muslims will be surrounded by loved ones if death is imminent. It is a sacred duty of the faithful to visit the sick, so hospitals should anticipate a large number of visitors. If possible, the Muslim patient should be moved to a side room to allow for the visitors. Since visitors may wish to help care for the sick, the health care providers may need to be prepared to articulate what care is best for the patient.

As death approaches, passages from the Qur'an are read and the shahadah, or declaration of belief in Allah, is recited. It is customary for prayers for forgiveness to be offered. Additionally, the patient may wish for his/her bed to be positioned so that his/her feet face Mecca.

Ideally, the last words a Muslim says will be the shahadah. At the time of death, those present may recite, "To Allah we belong and to Allah we return"—a phrase meant to hasten the departing soul on its journey to Allah.

Islam teaches that the soul of the deceased is freed from the body upon death. It is believed that the body will be resurrected after death, so it must be handled carefully. Health care providers should wear gloves while handling the body. If possible, providers should turn the patient's head toward Mecca, straighten the legs and arms, and close the mouth and eyes. Thereafter, the body should be covered with a clean, white cloth.

The health care providers should avoid washing the body when family is present, as this is traditionally done by a family member of the same sex. Customarily, the body is cleansed with scented water. Female bodies are traditionally dressed in five robes and males in three before a shroud is placed over the body. If the deceased visited Mecca, the sheets s/he wore during the hajj, a pilgrimage to Mecca required of all Muslims able to perform it, will sometimes be used as the shroud; this is not a frequent occurrence.

The family will most likely wish to pray in privacy before the body is taken to the morgue. Typically, the family will want the body released as quickly as possible so that the body can be prepared for burial. When buried, the body is placed in direct contact with the soil and the right side of the body is laid to face Mecca.

Most observant Muslim families will not allow a postmortem, as it is considered a desecration of the body and is thus haram, or forbidden. If a postmortem is absolutely necessary, great care should be taken to place all of the organs back into the body and to close all wounds, since it is believed that the body must be buried intact for resurrection to occur.

FOR MORE READING: ISLAM

Antes P. Medicine and the living tradition of Islam. In: Sullivan LE, ed. *Healing and Restoring: Health and Medicine in the World's Religious Traditions*. New York, NY: Macmillan. 1989: 173–202.

Hasan IY, Salaam Y. Faith and Islamic issues at the end of life. In: Puchalski CM, ed. *A Time for Listening and Caring: Spirituality and the Care of the Chronically Ill and Dying.*. Oxford, UK; Oxford University Press. 2006: 183–192.

Johnstone P. Medicine in Islam. In: Goodacre D, ed. *World Religions and Medicine*. 4th ed. Oxford, UK: Institute of Religion and Medicine.1983: 43–53.

Schott J, Henley A. Islam. In: Schott J, Henley A, eds. *Culture, Religion and Childbearing in a Multiracial Society*. Oxford, UK: Butterworth-Heinemann. 1996: 312–324.

4. Buddhism

••••

Overview FAQ

1. When, where, and how did Buddhism originate?

Buddhism originated in 528 BCE when a young man named Siddhartha Gautama (the historical *Buddha*) attained Enlightenment and began to teach in northeast India.

The Buddha came from royalty and was trained from a young age to succeed his father as king. After a secret excursion outside of the palace grounds exposed him to the suffering of others, he decided to dedicate himself to discovering the source of suffering and finding a way to end it.

At age 29, he left his wife and son behind to become a Hindu ascetic. After six years of yogic practices, the true nature of reality dawned on him as he meditated under a *bodhi* tree in Bodhgaya, India. He became known as the Awakened One (the Buddha) and began teaching others how to escape the earthly cycle of suffering.

2. Does Buddhism have sacred texts? What are they called?

The sacred texts of Buddhism are collectively called the *Dharma* and include:

- The *Pali* canon (the collected works of the Buddha);

- The *Tengyur* (the collected commentaries of Buddhist saints); and

- The *tantras* (the collected works of the founder and followers of the *Tantric* school of Buddhism).

The Buddha's teachings are divided into the *Sutras* (discourses on various topics), *Vinaya* (rules of conduct), and *Abhidharma* (philosophy).

In addition, any original teaching or commentary by a Buddhist master may become a central sacred text for that particular Buddhist tradition.

3. What are Buddhism's core beliefs?

The Buddha's fundamental teachings are the *Four Noble Truths*:

1. The experience of all living beings is wrought with suffering;

2. The cause of suffering is clinging to that which is subject to change;

3. Suffering ends when one relinquishes clinging and desire; and

4. Following the path to Enlightenment can end the cycle of suffering.

Buddhists believe in the law of cause and effect (*karma*) and reincarnation. As long as one continues to cling to this world, suffering will continue and that person will be trapped in a cycle of rebirth (*samsara*). When one attains Enlightenment (*Nirvana*), one is no longer bound by the cycle of reincarnation and suffering ends.

The way to achieve Enlightenment is by following the *Eightfold Path* of ethical behavior: right view—which means seeing the world through the lens of the Four Noble Truths—right intention, right speech, right action, right livelihood, right effort, right mindfulness, and right concentration.

4. What are Buddhism's core practices?

In terms of personal conduct, Buddhism emphasizes the Five Precepts: refraining from killing, stealing, harsh language or lying, sexual misconduct, and indulging in intoxicants.

Buddhist practice consists of contemplation of the Buddha's teachings and meditation in order to realize one's true nature. Meditation may be done in solitude or in regular meetings with other Buddhists. Depending on one's tradition, meditation can include the recitation of prayers and mantras, visualization of various emanations of the Buddha, and inducement of a trance-like state (*Samadhi*).

Compassionate activities, such as saving the lives of animals and helping those in need, are also encouraged. Violence is considered unwise and runs counter to the Four Noble Truths, since anger and violence imply an attachment to the material world.

5. What are Buddhism's important holidays? How are they celebrated?

Different Buddhist groups emphasize different holidays. Buddhist holidays follow the lunar calendar and will fall on different days each year. There are four main holidays celebrating different events in the life of the historical Buddha:

- **Chotrul** is a Tibetan celebration commemorating miracles performed by the historical Buddha during his lifetime on each of the first 15 days of the Lunar New Year (late February/early March). Many dedicate this time to prayer and meditation. The 15th day of the Lunar New Year is known as "The Day of Miracles," and many Buddhist monasteries host a ritual dance festival.

- **Wesak** (also called *Saga Dawa*): This holiday, which falls in May or June, celebrates the historical Buddha's birth, Enlightenment, and passing into Nirvana. The holiday includes a ceremonial feast and is dedicated to prayer and meditation.

- **Asala** (also called *Chokhor*): This holiday, which falls in July, celebrates the Buddha's first sermon, given to five disciples in seven weeks after his Enlightenment. Buddhists dedicate the day to reading and practicing the Buddha's teachings.

- **Lha Bab**: This holiday, which falls in November or December, celebrates one of the Buddha's "Eight Great Deeds" and his journey to heaven to repay his mother's kindness by teaching her and the celestial beings in heaven the path to Enlightenment. The holiday includes a ceremonial feast offering and is dedicated to prayer and meditation.

6. How many adherents of Buddhism are there in the United States? Are they located in a particular region?

There are estimated to be 6-7 million Buddhists living in the United States, of which 75% are of Asian decent. Western Buddhists are concentrated in the Northeast Corridor, Colorado, California, and the Pacific Northwest. Asian Buddhists are found primarily in major metropolitan areas nationwide.

7. What are the main sects or denominations within Buddhism?

For the first 400 years after his passing, the Buddha's disciples (many of them were ordained monks) carried on his tradition in small monasteries throughout Northern India. Shortly after the start of the Common Era, the tradition evolved into three main schools:

- **Mahayana** ("Great Vehicle") emphasizes the power of compassion to bring one to a state of Enlightenment. It also recognizes other Buddhist masters as being Buddhas in their own right. It is the most popular sect of Buddhism in China, India, Tibet, Vietnam, Japan, Korea, and Mongolia.

- **Theravada** ("Way of the Elders") focuses on traditional practices like meditation, and does not recognize latter-day Buddhas. It is the most popular sect of Buddhism in Sri Lanka, Myanmar, Thailand, Cambodia, Laos, Indonesia, Malaysia, and the Philippines.

- **Vajrayana** ("Diamond Vehicle") emphasizes mental and physical yogic techniques to move toward a natural state of Enlightenment. It is found most often in the Himalayas, Bhutan, Tibet, Nepal, and India.

Intersections with Health Care: FAQ

1. Does Buddhism have a particular view about what causes illness? Are there illness-related rituals?

Most Buddhists believe that illness is caused by one's past negative actions; as such, illness is also an opportunity to clear past debts. Many believe in holistic medicine and may prefer to use traditional herbal remedies and avoid Western medicine. Some sects of Buddhism also blame illness on malevolent spirits, requiring exorcism by a Buddhist master.

Many Buddhists will pray and perform rituals to the Medicine Buddha, a manifestation of the Buddha that promotes healing. Others may recite purification prayers, or try to create favorable circumstances for healing by engaging in virtuous deeds.

2. Does Buddhism prescribe a particular type of dress for men or women?

Ordained monks and nuns wear thin cotton robes of a specific hue according to their traditions; common colors include maroon, white, and orange. Lay Buddhists often dress modestly and may not be comfortable wearing shorts or revealing shirts.

Depending on the Buddhist denomination, believers may wear blessed cords or amulets around their necks or wrists. These items should not be removed without the patient's consent; if removal is necessary, they should be kept clean and safe.

3. Are there any prayer or ritual observances that are likely to occur during the patient's stay?

Prayer and meditation are core practices for almost all Buddhists. Depending on individual and denominational beliefs, these practices may occur throughout the day, with early morning being the most common time. Patients may prefer to meditate on the floor; some may also wish to sleep on the floor. Offer privacy and quiet during meditation; if possible, a side room should be made available.

Any scriptures in the room should be treated with great respect. Objects should not be placed on them, nor should they ever be placed on the floor.

Many Buddhists will choose to have an image of a Buddha in the room. This should not be touched without the patient's consent. Additionally, the patient may wish to have flowers or incense near the image. You may need to discuss these practices with the patient if, for example, incense is not allowed.

4. Does Buddhism have hygiene or washing requirements?

Most Buddhists wash their hands in running water before meditation. If access to running water is not an option, they should be provided with a jug or bowl.

5. Are there any dietary restrictions?

Many Buddhists are strict vegetarians and abstain from drinking alcohol or ingesting anything believed to dull the senses. However, the individual patient should be asked because there are no strict, universally observed dietary rules.

Most monks and nuns will not eat a meal after noon. On holidays, some lay Buddhists will also follow this practice. Others may choose to fast on new moon and full moon days.

6. Are there any medications, treatments, or procedures that Buddhists cannot accept?

One of the *Five Precepts* of Buddhist tradition calls for abstention from intoxicants that "cloud the mind," so some Buddhists are hesitant to take medication believed to alter their consciousness; this includes medicine that contains alcohol. Some may also prefer to meditate to ease pain before agreeing to begin taking pain medication. Vegetarians may wish to avoid medications containing animal byproducts.

7. Can Buddhist patients see providers of the opposite sex?

Most Buddhists do not have a religious conflict with seeing providers of the opposite sex.

8. Can Buddhists donate organs or accept donor organs?

Most Buddhists will not object to either organ donation or reception. However, there is no universal Buddhist teaching on this. Some view it as good karma to donate, while others believe that it disturbs the death process. In either case, no organs should be removed until consciousness has completely left the body (see question #13 below), as Buddhism teaches that consciousness exists within all organs of the body and not only in the brain.

9. Should I consult anyone other than the patient when seeking informed consent or other patient decisions?

In general, this is not necessary, although some patients may want the advice of a spiritual leader.

10. What is Buddhism's view on reproductive health and family planning? Are contraceptives okay? What about abortion? Voluntary sterilization?

Buddhism teaches that life begins at conception, so there is generally no objection to contraception that prevents fertilization (e.g., condoms).

Most Buddhists would consider abortion to be a very serious negative action, because Buddhism teaches that a fetus has consciousness either from the moment of conception or within several days of conception. However, there are a range of beliefs on this issue.

11. Are there particular beliefs or rituals concerning pregnancy and birth? What about postpartum women? What about women who have miscarried?

Depending on the branch of Buddhism, the family may choose to give their child a Buddhist name during a formal naming ceremony at the local temple or residence of a spiritual master. Before this ceremony, the child may be given an initial name by the parents. It is important to include both names in the clinical notes.

If a baby dies during delivery, a Buddhist clergy member will often be brought in to conduct rituals and pray. Lay Buddhists may also perform prayers and ceremonies for the recently deceased in the absence of a clergy member.

12. Are there end-of-life rituals or beliefs I need to know about?

For many Buddhists, it is important to have a clergy member around to guide them through the dying process. Most will also want to be surrounded by family and friends, who may chant mantras and meditate with the patient. Some may prefer to die in their own homes, and this should be allowed if possible.

Each denomination has slightly varying beliefs about the process of death, so each patient needs to be consulted. However, across all traditions, it is customary for Buddhists to spend their final time in meditation (both with loved ones and individually). In order to have an unclouded state of mind at death and pave the way for rebirth, some Buddhists resist sedatives or palliative drugs. Additionally, if an illness has advanced to an incurable stage, some Buddhist patients may refuse medical treatment.

If possible, the patient should be provided with a quiet space. Some may wish to have a Buddha figure close by and may burn incense or a candle.

Buddhism teaches that death is an inevitable part of the cycle of birth, death, and rebirth. Some Buddhist patients may resist life support, seeing it as interference to a natural cycle.

It is important to inform a fellow Buddhist of the death (including the time of death) so that proper prayers and rituals can be conducted for the recently deceased.

13. What should be done with the body after death?

Some Buddhists believe that consciousness remains in the body for up to three days after the patient stops breathing. It is important that the body not be moved or disturbed until consciousness ceases, if possible. If the patient dies in a hospital, the body should be left in an empty room where family and friends may gather to chant and pray. If no fellow Buddhists are present, staff should contact a Buddhist spiritual leader of the same denomination.

The body should be wrapped in a plain sheet with no religious symbols.

Most Buddhists will not object to a postmortem on religious grounds so long as it does not occur before the consciousness has left the body. Once consciousness has ceased, the body itself is not held in great reverence.

Generally, cremation is preferred.

· · · ·

Buddhism: Intersections with Health Care

Buddhism teaches that the body is a temporary shell for the spirit and should be treated with great respect so the mind can be free to concentrate on pursuing enlightenment, which is the ultimate goal of existence.

These beliefs have significant implications for practitioners of Western medicine. For example, some Buddhists believe that adversity can lead to personal transformation and transcendence; those who ascribe to this belief may resist some treatments or medications, especially those that cloud the mind. Similarly, aspects of modern Western health care facilities are at odds with a practicing Buddhist's needs. In particular, an ICU or emergency department—with bright lights, constant noise, and close patient monitoring—may not provide the quiet environment a Buddhist may need for contemplation and may be an additional source of stress. However, many Buddhists combine Western health care with Eastern cultural traditions.

Quick answers for many questions that arise when caring for a Buddhist patient may be found in the FAQ. For more in-depth explanations, consult the appropriate section below.

CAUSE OF ILLNESS AND HEALING RITUALS

Most Buddhists believe that illness is caused by one's past negative actions. The sum total of a person's actions, past and present, make up an individual's karma. A person's karma actively affects one's present and future experiences, thus making one responsible for one's own life. In Buddhism, therefore, an illness can be the culmination of many lifetimes' worth of karma. As such, it can be an opportunity to clear one's karmic debts.

Many Buddhists believe in holistic internal medicine and may see illness as a result of an imbalance in their inner energy channels. For this reason, some may prefer to take traditional herbal remedies and may choose to avoid Western medicine. Some Buddhists from Southeast Asia may also use traditional Indian or Chinese remedies. Thus, providers should always ask patients about any herbal or other remedies they are currently using. In addition, some sects of Buddhism may also blame illness on a malevolent spirit, requiring exorcism by a Buddhist master.

To treat an illness, many Buddhists will pray and perform rituals to the Medicine Buddha, a manifestation of the Buddha who promotes healing. Others may recite purification or obstacle-clearing prayers, or may try to create favorable circumstances (or positive karma) by engaging in virtuous deeds such as charitable giving or saving the life of an animal.

DRESS & MODESTY

Buddhism does not promulgate specific rules for how lay adherents should dress, and most followers will wear clothing that aligns with local culture.

Ordained monks and nuns wear thin cotton robes of a specific hue according to their countries of origin and Buddhist traditions; common colors include maroon, saffron (yellow), white, and orange. The robes are simple garments, draped around the body and over the shoulder, in emulation of the historical Buddha, Siddhartha Gautama, who is believed to have worn a patchwork robe made of donated cloth. Most robes are a single color, although Tibetan Buddhist robes are often more elaborate. Lay Buddhists often dress modestly and may not be comfortable wearing shorts or revealing shirts.

Depending on the Buddhist denomination, believers may wear blessed cords or amulets around their necks or wrist to ward off danger and promote good fortune. These items should not be removed without patient consent; if removal is necessary, they should be kept clean and safe.

PRAYER & RITUAL OBSERVANCES

Prayer and meditation are extremely important practices for almost all Buddhists, as it is through meditation that one comes to understand the Four Noble Truths and achieve enlightenment. Depending on individual and denominational beliefs, prayer and meditation may occur at any time throughout the day, with early morning being the most common time. Patients may prefer to meditate on the floor; some may also wish to sleep on the floor. Offer privacy and quiet during meditation to the extent it can be done; if possible, a side room should be made available.

There are a wide variety of meditation techniques employed by the various schools of Buddhist teaching. An adherent may just sit quietly, focus on breathing, engage in visualization, or contemplate a particular image, idea, or scriptural passage; some Buddhists may combine one or more methods. One of the most popular forms of meditation (particularly among Theravada Buddhists) is called *metta bhavana*. During metta bhavana or "loving-kindness," the practitioner aims to achieve a state of loving kindness toward all sentient beings.

Any scriptures in the room should be treated with great respect. Objects should not be placed on them, nor should they ever be placed on the floor.

Many Buddhists will choose to have an image of a Buddha in the room. This should not be touched without the patient's consent. Additionally, the patient may wish to have flowers or incense near the image. You may need to discuss these practices with the patient if, for example, incense is not allowed.

DIETARY REQUIREMENTS

Buddhism teaches non-violence and that a Buddhist should not cause the death of any other living being, so many Buddhists are strict vegetarians or vegans. Some may eat meat, but will limit the types of animal flesh they consume based on the amount of suffering and death involved. For example, eating beef may be permissible because many people can be fed from the death of a single cow; eating clams may be impermissible because many clams must be killed to make a single meal. Providers should discuss the nuances of dietary restrictions with Buddhist patients, although vegetarian meals are almost always safe.

Most monks and nuns will not eat a meal after noon, emulating the Buddha and following his recommendation. On holidays, some lay Buddhists will also follow this practice.

Some Buddhists may choose to fast on new moon and full moon days, to purify themselves, gain self-control, and help focus their minds. Depending on the school, fasting usually means abstaining from all solid foods but *not* liquids; in addition, fasts often begin after noon. Furthermore, although some fasting is encouraged, asceticism is not; the Buddha taught moderation in all things. Thus, a fast may have less impact for a Buddhist patient on a regimen of drug therapy than it might for a Muslim patient for whom fasting requires total abstention from all liquids and solids.

Many Buddhists also abstain from drinking alcohol or ingesting anything that would dull the senses, pollute the body, and affect one's mindfulness. As noted below, medications containing alcohol or narcotics should be avoided when possible. If a physician does prescribe medication containing alcohol or narcotics, the nature of and reason for the prescription should be carefully explained to the patient. This prohibition is not a hard and fast rule followed by all, and the individual patient should always be consulted.

MEDICATION, TREATMENT, OR PROCEDURE RESTRICTIONS

One of the Five Precepts of Buddhist tradition states that adherents are to abstain from intoxicants that cloud the mind. Therefore, some Buddhists may be hesitant to take medication that is believed to alter their state of consciousness, including medicines that contain either alcohol or narcotics. Some may also prefer to meditate to ease pain before they decide to begin taking medication.

If a particular medication for pain-relief purposes can affect the mind, providers should discuss alternate methods of pain relief with the patient. However, if a medication is necessary to resolve an illness, providers should clearly explain what they are recommending and why. It may also be helpful for the patient to speak to his/her Buddhist spiritual leader, who may be a Buddhist master, monk, nun, or revered layperson, depending on the branch of Buddhism practiced and the individual beliefs of the patient.

Some Buddhists are vegetarian and may not want to take medications that contain animal byproducts (see Dietary Requirements).

GENDER & MODESTY

In general, Buddhists do not believe that there is a religious conflict with seeing providers of the opposite sex. However, this may vary depending on culture or country of origin; each patient should be consulted for his/her preferences.

ORGAN DONATION

Most Buddhists will not object either to organ donation or reception. However, there is no universal Buddhist teaching on this, and there is some disagreement among the different Buddhist schools.

Some schools view it as good karma to donate organs, as giving the gift of life to another is a tremendous act of kindness and manifestation of metta, loving-kindness.

Others believe that organ donation disturbs the death process, or that issues of life and death should be left to take their natural course.

In either case, no organs should be removed until consciousness has completely left the body (see End of Life). Buddhism teaches that consciousness exists within all organs of the body and not only in the brain. Thus, one does not assume that a person is dead because brain function has ceased. Indeed, it may be necessary for a religious leader to confirm death before a family will allow organs to be harvested.

INFORMED CONSENT & PATIENT DECISION MAKING

There is no overarching rule on decision making; the patient should be asked whether or not s/he desires a spiritual leader to be brought into the conversation. Depending on the branch of Buddhism practiced and the individual preference of the patient, the spiritual leader may be a Buddhist master, a monk, nun, or revered clergyperson. Some Buddhists may also wish for respected family members to be present when discussing important decisions.

REPRODUCTIVE HEALTH & FAMILY PLANNING

Generally, Buddhism does not prescribe or condemn particular sexual partnerships in the way many other religious traditions do (e.g., Christianity, Judaism, or Islam, all of which frown upon sex outside of marriage), nor does it teach monogamy. As long as the relationships themselves are entered into freely and are not dependent on lying or manipulation, all manner of relationships may be permissible. This includes homosexual as well as heterosexual relationships. Some Buddhists may also practice chastity in order to focus and devote more energy to reaching enlightenment.

While there are no established doctrines around family planning for Buddhists, there is a general reluctance to disturb the natural development of life. As a result, some Buddhists will accept all methods of family planning, but with varying degrees of reluctance. Generally, Buddhism teaches that life begins at conception, so there is not likely to be an objection to contraceptives that prevent conception (e.g., a condom). Conversely, those that would prevent a fertilized ovum from being successfully implanted (e.g., an intrauterine device or emergency contraception) may be more problematic.

Most Buddhists would consider abortion to be a very serious, negative action because it is taught that the fetus has consciousness either at the moment of conception or within several days thereafter. Some Buddhists will make allowances for the health of the mother, arguing that the mother's life takes precedence over fetal health. Each individual should be asked, however, because there are a wide range of beliefs. Depending on the circumstances, it may also be helpful to involve a Buddhist spiritual leader in the conversation.

PREGNANCY & BIRTH

Given that a sentient being has the capacity to be reborn into many forms, both human and animal, human birth is generally viewed as auspicious. A baby is considered particularly fortunate if it is born with all six senses. In Buddhism, these are: taste, touch, smell, hearing, sight, and mental functioning. Any disabilities with which a child might be born are often attributed to karma, and are regarded as the consequences of negative actions in a past life.

Depending on the branch of Buddhism, the family may choose to give their child a Buddhist name during a formal naming ceremony at the local temple or residence of a spiritual master. Before this ceremony, the child may be given an interim name by the parents. It is important to include both names in the clinical notes, if the second name is already chosen. In some schools, the naming ceremony occurs later in life (anywhere from three to eight years of age).

If a baby dies during delivery, a Buddhist clergy member will often be brought in to conduct rituals and prayers for the dead. Lay Buddhists may also perform prayers and ceremonies for the recently deceased in the absence of a clergy member.

END OF LIFE

Buddhism teaches that death is inevitable and a part of the cycle of birth, death, and rebirth. Although the physical body will pass away, the essence of the person's consciousness will be reborn into another vessel (unless the patient has reached enlightenment). Death is a necessary part of this process. Because of this, some Buddhist patients may resist life support and resuscitation, seeing it as needlessly interfering with a natural process.

A Buddhist who knows that s/he is near death will probably spend a great deal of time in meditation, necessitating as much peace and quiet as can be provided.

For many Buddhists, it is important to have a clergy member present to guide them through the dying process. Most will also want to be surrounded by family and friends, who may chant mantras and meditate with the patient; for many Buddhists, one of the greatest acts of kindness is to help another person attain a positive state of mind in preparation for death. Some believe that Buddhist tradition dictates that people not cry in the presence of a dying person or someone who has ceased to breathe; it is believed that this may disturb consciousness and clarity of mind at the moment of death. Some Buddhists may prefer to die in their own homes, which should be allowed if possible.

Each denomination has slightly varying beliefs about the process of death, so each patient and family should be consulted. However, across the traditions, it is customary for Buddhists to spend their final time in meditation as much as they are able (both with loved ones and individually), given the importance of one's state of mind at the moment of death. In order to have a clear, unclouded state of mind at death, which influences one's rebirth, some Buddhists may resist sedatives or palliative care drugs. Additionally, if illness has advanced to an incurable stage, some Buddhist patients may refuse medical treatment.

If possible, the patient should be provided with a quiet space. Some may wish to have a Buddha figure close by and may use a candle or burn incense. If this is not allowed in a specific facility, explain the policy to the patient's family and offer alternatives (e.g., a small lamp placed on the bedside table).

As noted above, for Buddhists, death is not necessarily synonymous with lack of brain function. Many Buddhists believe that a person's consciousness exists in all the organs in addition to the brain, so death occurs when life has left all the organs. A Buddhist spiritual leader may need to be consulted to determine when a patient is dead; this is especially important if the patient or family has consented to organ donation.

Some Buddhists believe that consciousness remains in the body for up to three days after the patient stops breathing. It may be very important to the family that the body not be moved or disturbed until consciousness ceases. This may be impossible in a hospital, in which case hospital policy should be explained to the family and alternatives explored. An alternative could be moving the entire hospital bed into the morgue while leaving the body itself untouched. If the patient takes his/her final breath in the hospital, the body should be left in an empty room, where family and friends may gather to chant and read prayers.

If no fellow Buddhists are present at the time of death, a Buddhist spiritual leader of the same denomination as the patient should be contacted. It is also important to inform a fellow Buddhist of the death (including the time of death) so that proper prayers and rituals to benefit the recently deceased can be conducted.

The body should be wrapped in a plain sheet with no religious symbols. Most Buddhists will not object to a postmortem on religious grounds so long as it does not occur before consciousness has left the body. Once consciousness has ceased, Buddhists may be quite willing to allow postmortems because the body itself is not held in great reverence thereafter. It is important that the health care provider know the individual's beliefs before death so that they are respected. Generally, cremation is preferred.

FOR MORE READING: BUDDHISM

Arond DE. Eye on religion: Buddhism and medicine. *Southern Med J*. 2006; 99[12]: 1450-51.

Birnbaum R. Chinese Buddhist traditions of healing and the life cycle. In: Sullivan LE, ed. *Healing and Restoring: Health and Medicine in the World's Religious Traditions*. New York, NY: Macmillian. 1989: 33-57.

Pye M. Suffering and health in Mahayana Buddhism. In: Goodacre D., ed. *World Religions and Medicine*. 4th ed. Oxford, UK: Institute of Religion and Medicine. 1983: 25-31.

Rapgay L. A Buddhist approach to end-of-life care. In: Puchalski CM, ed. *A Time for Listening and Caring: Spirituality and the Care of the Chronically Ill and Dying*. Oxford, UK: Oxford University Press. 2006: 131-37.

5. Hinduism

Overview FAQ

1. When, where, and how did Hinduism originate?

Hinduism began as a highly localized religion on the Indian subcontinent. In contrast to many other religious traditions, there is no single date or particular place where the religion was founded, nor is there a singular founder. Instead, Hinduism recognizes many teachers and prophets, each of whom are believed to have had direct contact with a higher power.

Hinduism is an amalgamation of numerous cultures and practices that evolved over time. Historically and culturally, the religion's roots can be traced to ancient civilizations and religions in India, Pakistan, Afghanistan, Turkmenistan, and other countries on the Indian subcontinent. It is generally accepted to be the oldest organized religion in the world, dating to circa 3000 BCE.

2. Does Hinduism have sacred texts? What are they called?

Unlike many other religions, what is considered a sacred text may vary from believer to believer. However, three of the major Hindu scriptures widely accepted as authoritative are the *Vedas*, the *Bhagavad Gita*, and the *Upanishads*. The Vedas are believed to be divinely revealed eternal wisdom, and the Bhagavad Gita is often considered to be a summary of Hindu spiritual teachings. The Upanishads focus on meditation, the nature of God, and philosophy.

3. What are the core beliefs of Hinduism?

Hinduism does not have a single system of morality, a prescribed theological system, or an organizational hierarchy. Rather, the Hindu life is reflected in a variety of beliefs and practices. It is thus sometimes perceived as more of a way of life than a set of universal dogmas.

Though a wide range of beliefs characterize the religion, most Hindus believe that there is one ultimate reality behind the universe that cannot be fully grasped by humans. There are also various gods and goddesses that are manifestations of different characteristics of this ultimate reality. Individual practitioners may focus worship on or exult one particular deity. For example, the commonly worshipped gods *Brahma*, *Shiva*, and *Vishnu* represent the creative, destructive, and sustaining powers of the ultimate reality and each has its own sect of worshippers.

The majority of Hindus believe that the soul (*atman*) is eternal and reincarnated. Each individual goes through a cycle of birth, death, and rebirth (*samsara*) governed by a law of cause and effect (*karma*). The ultimate goal of a believer's life is to liberate oneself (*moksha*) from this cycle of rebirth through the realization of one's identity with the ultimate reality.

There is no singular way that one achieves *moksha*, but rather each individual chooses a discipline (*yoga*), and path (*marga*), which becomes his/her religious life (*dharma*).

4. What are the core practices of Hinduism?

The vast majority of Hindus engage in religious rituals every day. Many pray at sunrise and before sunset; some may also choose to pray at midday. Those who are able may wash and put on clean clothes before praying to purify themselves. It is common for Hindu homes to contain a small shrine with statues and pictures of Hindu gods; this becomes the place where family members in the house worship. Worship may involve recitation from religious scriptures, meditation, singing hymns, or chanting mantras. There is also an elaborate set of rituals based around important life events such as birth, marriage, and death.

Hindus may also follow the teachings of a particular sect or Hindu *guru* ("teacher"). For example, many Hare Krishna practitioners follow strict rules barring recreational drugs and intoxicants (including caffeine); meat, fish, and eggs; gambling; and sexual relations outside procreation within marriage. In terms of *Vaishnavas* (those who worship Vishnu), practitioners may avoid certain foods, like onions, garlic, and mushrooms because of their purportedly negative effects on one's consciousness.

5. What are Hinduism's important holidays? How are they celebrated?

Hindu festivals occur throughout the year in accordance with the Hindu calendar, which is based on solar and lunar movements. Depending on the particular group of believers, different festivals are emphasized. Most celebrations involve a visit to the temple and fasting.

Three of the most frequently observed festivals are: *Diwali*, *Holi*, and *Maha Shivratri*.

- **Diwali** is the most widely celebrated Hindu holiday, and lasts for several days in late October or early November. It is considered by many Hindus to be the start of a new year. Diwali is the "festival of lights," and celebrates the triumph of light (good and knowledge) over darkness (evil and ignorance). For Diwali, many Hindus wear new clothes, share food, light firecrackers, burn small oil lamps, and give presents to their gods (i.e., the particular manifestations of the divine that they worship).

- **Holi**, which occurs over a period of two to five days in February or March, is a festival of colors that celebrates creation and renewal. It is most commonly associated with the stories of a god of creation (Vishnu), one of his incarnations (*Krishna*), and the defeat of a demoness (*Holika*). Traditionally, people throw colored powder, water, dye, or paint at each other during this celebration.

⤖ **Maha Shivratri** is celebrated in February or March and is dedicated to the god Shiva, a god of transformation/destruction. On this day, Hindus may spend the night at a temple worshipping Shiva, offering milk, and fasting.

6. How many adherents of Hinduism are there in the United States? Are they located in a particular region?

There are approximately 1.5 million Hindus in the United States. The states with the largest Hindu populations are California, New York, New Jersey, Texas, and Illinois. This includes converts to Hinduism, such as Hare Krishnas.

There are also millions of yoga practitioners worldwide. Yoga is an integral part of life for many Hindus, but is not solely a Hindu practice.

7. What are the main sects or denominations within Hinduism?

Hinduism has no central authority or hierarchy, no single founder, and no single holy book. As such, Hinduism includes a wide diversity of beliefs and practices. Acceptance of the diversity of ways to live a religious life is fundamental to the Hindu belief system.

Although there is tremendous diversity, it is not limitless. There are sects of Hindus, many based on worshipping a particular god or goddess (e.g., Vaishnavas, who worship Vishnu, or *Saivas,* who worship Siva). The Hare Krishna movement is also considered a subset of Hinduism.

• • • •

Intersections with Health Care: FAQ

1. Does Hinduism have a particular view about what causes illness? Are there illness-related rituals?

Hinduism generally attributes illness to karma; illness, accidents, and injuries are believed to be caused by past poor behavior. Since karma accrues over many lifetimes, illness may be a result of one's actions in either this or a past life.

Some Hindus use alternative medicine like *Ayurveda,* a traditional Indian medical system that relies on diet, meditation, and herbal/natural remedies. Ayurvedic practitioners are called *vaids,* and patients may wish to consult them before or in conjunction with Western medical treatment.

2. Does Hinduism prescribe a particular type of dress for men or women?

Many Hindu women prefer modest dress. Some women wear a traditional Indian garment called a *sari,* a long cloth wrapped around the waist and over the shoulder and worn over a short blouse and underskirt. These women may prefer longer hospital gowns that are fully closed in the back. Many Hindu women also wear a small colored spot (*bindi* or *chandlo*) on their foreheads. Traditionally, this indicates that they are married. Married women may also wear a streak of vermilion powder (*sindur*) in the part of their hair, as well as a gold marriage necklace or bracelet; these should not be removed unless necessary.

Many Hindu men also dress modestly, preferring to wear a long shirt over loose pajama-style trousers. Traditionally, men also wear a sacred thread draped over the shoulder or tied around the wrist, which should not be removed if possible. If removal is necessary, the thread should be saved for the patient and never be placed on the floor, near feet or shoes, or in a place that may be contaminated by bodily fluids.

3. Are there any prayer or ritual observances that are likely to occur during the patient's stay?

Most devout Hindus pray three times a day: at sunrise, noon and sunset. Prayer usually involves recitation of a mantra and is done facing north or east; some Hindus also wash themselves before prayer. Prayer should not be disturbed by staff unless necessary.

Some Hindus may wish to have religious icons, candles, statues of a family deity, a bell, or food by their bedside. These items should be treated respectfully and handled only with consent.

4. Does Hinduism have hygiene or washing requirements?

Personal cleanliness is deeply important in Hinduism, and many Hindu patients will wish to bathe daily. Washing the hands is considered essential before and after meals, and prior to prayer. Additionally, a patient may want to rinse out his/her mouth after eating.

Running water is preferred for cleansing. If the patient has limited mobility, a bowl of water should be offered.

Additionally, Hindu tradition teaches that the right hand is used for "clean" tasks and the left for "unclean" tasks. Important items and food should not be offered from the left hand.

5. Are there any dietary restrictions?

Most Hindus do not consume beef or pork, and some may not eat chicken, eggs, or fish. Dairy is generally acceptable, as long as it is free of animal fat. However, some Hindus are strict vegetarians and will consume neither foods containing meat or meat byproducts, nor eat from plates that have come into contact with prohibited foods. In a hospital, many would prefer entirely vegetarian food or food brought from home rather than hospital food.

It is common for some Hindus to consume milk, yogurt, butter, *ghee* (clarified butter), and fruit during illness, as these are considered to promote purity and harmony. Additionally, some Hindus believe that certain foods have healing or harmful qualities. During treatment, it can be a good idea to discuss diet along with medication so these issues can come to the surface.

Some Hindus may fast on certain holidays. Generally, the sick can be excused from fasting.

6. Are there any medications, treatments, or procedures that Hindus cannot accept?

Taking medication is generally avoided as much as possible because Western medicines are believed to cloud the mind and pollute the body. Thus, Hindu patients may be resistant to various treatments including more aggressive ones. Additionally, the patient may be using ayurvedic or other homeopathic treatments; providers should be sure to ask about these. Patients may also wish to avoid medication that contains animal products if possible.

7. Can Hindus see providers of the opposite sex?
Modesty is important for most Hindus (and especially women), and female patients often prefer female doctors. If a same-sex doctor is not available, a chaperone may be necessary. It is customary for a young woman to be accompanied by her mother or sister (or possibly her father or brother) and for a married woman to be accompanied by her husband or sister-in-law.

8. Can Hindus donate organs or accept donor organs?
There are generally no objections to giving or receiving organ donations. However, some Hindus may be more willing to donate certain less-essential organs (e.g., the corneas) over others (e.g., the heart). Others object to organ donation altogether, because they view it as interfering with the cycle of birth and rebirth (samsara).

9. Should I consult anyone other than the patient when seeking informed consent or other patient decisions?
In many cases, it is prudent to involve the family in matters of diagnosis and treatment. Traditionally, a family elder is the spokesperson. More traditional Hindus will also seek permission of a husband or father before consenting to treatment for a female patient.

10. What are Hinduism's views on reproductive health and family planning? Are contraceptives okay? What about abortion? Voluntary sterilization?
There are no prescribed Hindu teachings on birth control. However, there is often strong social pressure on Hindu women to give birth. In most cases, the husband prefers to be included in any discussions about contraception or sterilization. However, men may refuse to undergo any fertility tests, because women are traditionally considered the cause of infertility.

Contraceptive methods that can cause spotting or irregular periods may be unacceptable because some women's activities (both religious and in the household) may be restricted when she menstruates (a time when Hindu women are traditionally regarded as unclean). Women may also avoid gynecological exams during menstruation.

Abortion is traditionally frowned upon, but there is a great deal of variance within the religion. When the mother's life is in danger, many women believe that her health takes precedence over the fetus. Some Hindus also feel that it is more acceptable to abort a female fetus, given the high value Indian society places on males, although this is uncommon in the United States.

11. Are there particular beliefs or rituals concerning pregnancy and birth? What about postpartum women? What about women who have miscarried?
Though there are many Hindu customs surrounding pregnancy and childbirth, they vary tremendously among families, communities, and geographical areas.

Bathing may be an issue for new mothers; they may wait to bathe until a religious bath can be performed. In some communities, a female close to the new mother symbolically washes the mother's breasts before she feeds her baby for the first time.

Many mothers do not feel comfortable with their babies being kept in a separate room, so communication between the patient and staff is recommended if an infant must be moved to a nursery or NICU. Mothers may also be uncomfortable if infants are bathed without their consent.

Some Hindus perform a welcome ceremony for the baby. This ceremony includes writing "om," a sacred sound, on the baby's tongue with honey or ghee (clarified butter); because honey is not recommended for infants due to the risk of infant botulism, providers may need to discuss alternatives with parents. Hymns, mantras, and the name of God are whispered into the baby's ear, and some families wrap the baby in a religiously significant cloth. If a family performs this ceremony in the hospital, then privacy is appreciated when possible.

The mother may receive a large number of visitors, since birth is a cause for great celebration and extended family is generally expected to visit.

Some Hindu parents will want to know the exact time of birth so that they can get an accurate horoscope; the first letter of the baby's name is often chosen by the astrologist. The full name is usually chosen by an elder or priest on the tenth day after birth.

According to traditional Hindu belief, the soul enters the fetus during the seventh month of pregnancy. Thus, many families may wish to perform a proper religious funeral if a miscarriage occurs after this period. Some Hindus believe that miscarriage is the karmic fault of the mother, and extra emotional support may be necessary for the woman.

In the case of stillbirth, the body should be wrapped in a towel or clean, white cloth and made available for the family to view.

12. Are there end-of-life rituals or beliefs I need to know about?

Most Hindus prefer to die in their own homes, so death in the hospital may be very distressing for patient and family alike. If a terminal patient must remain in the hospital, staff should be prepared for a potentially large number of visitors; the space provided and visiting hours may require some adjustment. A dying patient may also request to be placed on the ground during his/her final breaths to be closer to the earth.

The family should be consulted to see if they wish to perform the Hindu Last Rites in the hospital; a *pundit* (priest) may be brought in to administer them. Last Rites often include readings from the Bhagavad Gita, or, for a foreign-born patient, a text with meaning in the patient's original language, such as Gujarati or Tamil, and tying of a thread around the patient's wrist or neck, marking the forehead with blessed dust, sprinkling the patient with water from the Ganges, or placing a sacred *tulsi* leaf (basil) in the patient's mouth. Additionally, the family may bring money and clothes for the patient to touch so that they can be distributed to the needy in the patient's name after death.

Traditionally, Hinduism teaches that the dying person should concentrate his/her mind on a personal mantra to create the proper state of mind for reincarnation. If the patient is unconscious, a family member may chant a mantra in the person's right ear.

13. What should be done with the body after death?

Some Hindu families are extremely concerned with who touches the body after death. If no family members are available, observe the following guidelines when possible: Do not remove sacred items like threads or jewelry from the body. Consult the family before touching the body; if it is necessary to touch the body, use of gloves is appreciated. Close the patient's eyes, straighten his/her limbs, and wrap the body in a plain sheet. Do not cut nails or trim hair without consent. In most cases, the body should not be washed; cleansing is part of Hindu funeral rites and will usually be carried out by relatives. If a body must be left in a room overnight, a light or candle should be left burning and the body placed with the head pointing north and the feet south. If the family requests a viewing, staff should try to ensure that the room is free of any non-Hindu religious symbols.

Most Hindus will not allow a postmortem unless it is legally required, because opening the body is believed to be disrespectful to the dead and his/her family. If one is necessary, the patient's family will most likely insist that all organs be returned to the body for cremation (all Hindus over age five are cremated).

If possible, less than 24 hours should elapse before the funeral, and the death certificate should be filled out as quickly as possible. Traditionally, when an adult dies, the eldest son is responsible for making funeral arrangements. If the body remains at the hospital for more than a day, it is likely that extended family and friends will visit to pay their last respects.

• • • •

Hinduism: Intersections with Health Care

What we call "Hinduism" actually refers to a rich variety of religious beliefs and practices: Hinduism is an umbrella term for a religion that was formed by the amalgamation of many smaller, local faiths. It does not have a single founder, founding date, or creed. The name Hindu historically referred to people from the area near the Indus River, within the borders of India, Tibet, Nepal, and Pakistan. Until the 20th century, Hinduism was largely confined to that area; today, Hindus are found worldwide.

Along with the tremendous diversity within Hinduism, there is also tremendous local variation. People from two different villages in the same region might practice very differently (although many of these differences are matters of culture, more than specifically religious). This can make it very difficult to generalize about what a particular patient might need, making good communication all the more important.

Despite the infinite variations in practice, there are some shared beliefs and rituals. In general, most Hindus see healing as a holistic process meant to encourage health and well-being in mind and body.

Quick answers for many questions that arise when caring for a Hindu patient may be found in the FAQ. For more in-depth explanations, consult the appropriate section below.

ILLNESS: BELIEFS AND RITUALS

Hindus often attribute illness to karma (the law of cause and effect). Illness, accidents, and injuries are believed to be the result of one's past bad actions, and become means by which one may be purified. Although an immediate cause may be recognized (e.g., food poisoning caused by something one ate), the larger, karmic cause is also acknowledged.

In addition, the majority of Hindus believe that the soul (atman) is eternal. Each individual goes through a cycle of birth, death, and rebirth (samsara). Since karma is believed to accrue over multiple lifetimes, an illness may be a result of one's actions in either this life or a past one.

Hinduism does not have a single system of morality, prescribed theological system, or organizational hierarchy. Despite this variance, the vast majority of Hindus engage in religious rituals every day. Many pray at sunrise, midday, and before sunset. Frequently, those that are ill pray more often, and chant mantras as many times as possible throughout the day; it is believed that through these prayers and mantras, one may become healthier. Additionally, a patient's loved ones may offer prayers to strengthen the ill individual.

In addition to prayer, some Hindus may want to use traditional medical systems such as Ayurveda. Ayurveda is a traditional Indian system of medicine that treats imbalances in the body with diet, exercise, meditation, and herbal remedies. In Ayurveda, there are three "bodily humors" (*doshas*) which regulate mind-body harmony:

- *Vata* (wind) governs movement, including breathing, blood flow, and the elimination of waste;

- *Pitta* (bile) governs heat, metabolism, and transformation; and

- *Kapha* (phlegm) heals wounds, lubricates joints, moisturizes the skin, and regulates the immune system.

Imbalance in any of these areas (either because of improper consumption of food or the presence of evil spirits) may be identified as the cause of illness. Practitioners of Ayurveda are called *vaids* in the Hindi language, and may be consulted before the patient seeks Western medical treatment. Providers should ask whether a patient practices Ayurveda and what herbal remedies, if any, s/he is currently using.

DRESS & MODESTY

Many Hindu women prefer modest dress. Those who keep with the traditional dressing customs of India often wear a sari, which is a long piece of fabric wrapped around the torso, neck, and shoulders, and worn over a short blouse and an underskirt. Many women who wear saris prefer long gowns that are closed in the back and night dresses; if long hospital gowns are unavailable, they may want to wear a dressing gown or shawl. Most Hindu men also dress modestly, preferring to wear a long shirt over pajamas, although most men in the United States wear Western-style clothing.

Many Hindu women also wear a small colored spot (called a bindi or chandlo) on their foreheads. Traditionally, this indicates that they are married and is symbolic of the bond between a wife and her husband (historically, the mark was made on a bride using the groom's blood). Widows sometimes wear a black bindi, while younger unmarried women may wear a bindi that matches their clothes. A married or widowed woman may become upset if the bindi needs to be removed; providers should not remove the bindi without getting the patient's consent and explaining clearly the reasons for removal.

Married women may also wear a red streak of vermilion powder (sindur) in the part of their hair. Some Hindu women in the hospital may wish to apply their bindi and sindur every morning, and may require some assistance with this.

Hindu women traditionally wear a gold marriage necklace or bangle, which should not be removed unless absolutely necessary. Other marriage jewelry may include nose rings, toe rings, and earrings.

Some Hindu men wear a sacred thread; it is usually draped over the shoulder, and sometimes tied around the wrist, which also should also not be removed without consent and explanation. They receive this cord at a ceremony marking their transition from puberty to adulthood; it also symbolizes ritual purity. Some men may also wear a ring or amulet which has been blessed by a priest. If removal of either of these items is necessary, patient consent should be obtained. Once the items are removed, they should never be placed on the floor, near feet or shoes, or in a place that may be contaminated by bodily fluids.

GENDER & MODESTY

Modesty is important for most Hindus. Female patients generally prefer female doctors. If a doctor of the same sex cannot be provided, then a chaperone may be necessary. It is customary for a young woman to be accompanied by her mother or sister (or possibly her father or brother) and for a married woman to be accompanied by her husband or sister-in-law.

In inpatient settings, some Hindu women may prefer to be in same-gender wards if they are available.

PRAYER & RITUAL OBSERVANCES

Most devout Hindus pray three times a day (at sunrise, noon, and sunset); those that are sick may pray more often. Prayer often involves the recitation of a mantra and is preferably done facing north or east. It is customary to wash oneself for purification before prayer, so accommodation for this cleansing should be provided; purification and washing are key Hindu tenets (see Hygiene & Washing Requirements). Prayer should not be disturbed by staff unless necessary.

In addition to daily prayer, many Hindus perform *puja*. Puja are demonstrations of reverence for the divine done through song and prayer; they are believed to bring the individual or family closer to the family deity. Puja also often involve offerings of food, incense, and flowers to a statue or image of the god. The food is eaten at the end of the ritual. As incense and open flames will not be allowed in a medical setting, it is unlikely that a patient will expect to perform a formal puja while hospitalized. However, family or friends may bring food from home, and providers may need to ensure that the food is acceptable given the patient's medical state.

Some Hindus may wish to have religious icons, candles, a statue of the family deity, a bell, or traditional food by their bedsides, either for use in prayer or puja or simply as a source of comfort. These items should be treated respectfully and handled only after consulting the patient.

HYGIENE & WASHING REQUIREMENTS

Personal cleanliness is very important to most Hindus, and most Hindus will want to bathe daily as well as prior to meals and prayer if possible. Many will prefer a shower to a bath, as running water is considered more pure than standing water, and may want to wash their hair as well as their bodies. If a shower is unavailable or is not feasible, ask the patient if s/he would like to use a jug to pour water and simulate the movement of water in a shower.

Most Hindus will also want to wash after going to the bathroom. Running water or a jug of water should be provided in the same room as the toilet; a bidet is ideal. If a patient needs a bedpan, a bowl of water should be offered afterward and a health care provider (ideally of the same sex) should assist the patient with washing. This may be a delicate issue for some older Indians, who may not be accustomed to Western-style toilets.

Washing one's hands is considered essential before and after meals and prior to prayer. The patient should also be able to rinse his/her mouth after eating.

Additionally, Hindu tradition teaches that the right hand is used for "clean" tasks and the left for "unclean" tasks. Important items and food should not be offered from the left hand.

DIETARY REQUIREMENTS

Hinduism has a great deal to say about diet. Along with some forbidden foods, Hinduism also believes that some foods have healing or harmful properties.

Most Hindus believe that it is a religious requirement to avoid doing harm to any living creature; thus, many Hindus are sensitive to their food sources and are vegetarians. In addition, cows are considered to be a holy symbol of the gods' bounty, so almost all Hindus avoid beef and beef products. Pork is generally also avoided, as pigs are believed to be unclean. In a hospital, many would prefer entirely vegetarian food or food brought from home rather than hospital food.

Other than avoiding beef and pork, there are a variety of interpretations of Hindu dietary requirements. Some may not eat chicken, eggs, or fish. Dairy is generally acceptable, as long as it is free of animal fat (e.g., cheese is only acceptable if rennet-free, and ice cream may contain animal fat). Some Hindus are strict vegetarians who will not consume any food from a plate that has come into contact with prohibited foods/utensils or that has been prepared in the same kitchen where meat is cooked.

If there are no medical dietary restrictions, patients should be allowed to bring food from home. It is common for some Hindus to consume milk, yogurt, butter, ghee (clarified butter), and fruits during illness, as they are considered to be foods which promote purity and harmony. *Prashad*, a food commonly given to those in poor health, is made of milk, yogurt, ghee, honey, and sugar that has been blessed and offered to the family gods.

Many Hindus may practice fasting or food restriction of one type or another, although there is no specific prescription for fasting in Hinduism. Some practitioners also choose to fast during times of illness in an attempt to return harmony to the body. Some fasting patients may still accept milk, tea, fruit, and/or yogurt. Generally, the sick can be excused from fasting, but the patient should be consulted, especially if a fast will hinder treatment or recovery.

Additionally, some Hindus believe that certain foods have healing or harmful qualities. These foods are characterized as either hot or cold, good or bad, or auspicious or inauspicious, and are believed to either aid or hamper recovery. For example, those suffering from a lung infection may avoid milk because it is considered wet and cold. Coconut is also considered a sacred food, and ayurvedic treatments may require eating or avoiding certain foods at certain times.

As a general rule, it is a good idea to discuss diet alongside medication for Hindu patients so issues like these may come to the surface.

MEDICATION, TREATMENT, AND PROCEDURE RESTRICTIONS

Many Hindus feel that Western medicine tends to overmedicate the patient, especially in the use of antibiotics. Some are also hesitant to seek medical treatment because they see Western medicine's focus on treating the specific illness (rather than treating the person as a whole) as dehumanizing.

Taking medications is generally avoided as much as possible because they may cloud the mind, pollute the body, and distance the soul from the divine. Thus, Hindu patients may be resistant to aggressive treatments. Additionally, the patient may be practicing Ayurveda; health care practitioners should ask Hindu patients if they are using ayurvedic or homeopathic remedies before starting other treatments.

Some Hindus believe that an animal killed for medicine might have been a person in another life; in addition, there is a strong injunction against harming other living creatures. Therefore, taking any medications with animal products is believed to bring bad karma. If possible, avoid medication that contains animal products, including capsules that are made using beef or pork products.

ORGAN DONATION

There are generally no objections to giving or receiving organ donations. *Daan*, selfless giving, is one of the 10 virtuous acts a Hindu can perform. Since a donor organ can help save the life of another, it is an acceptable act. There may, however, be a concern that some of the donor's karma will accompany the organ into its new body; there is a belief that the recipient may take on some of the characteristics of the donor. There is also a concern for the donor's afterlife and reincarnation, since part of the donor will continue to live in the recipient.

Some Hindus may be more willing to donate certain less-essential organs (e.g., the corneas) over others (e.g., the heart). Others object to organ donation altogether, because they view it as interfering with the cycle of birth and rebirth (samsara).

These concerns do not extend to giving blood, because the soul is believed to exist only in the organs, so blood transfusions are allowed.

INFORMED CONSENT & PATIENT DECISION MAKING

In most cases, it is essential to involve the family in matters of diagnosis, treatment, consent for procedures, etc. Traditionally, in most Hindu families an elder in the family is a spokesperson, and his/her consent and involvement should be respected.

For female patients, it is customary for traditional Hindus to seek the permission of the woman's husband or father before signing a consent form. However, as with all patients, the individual beliefs of the woman need to be respected.

REPRODUCTIVE HEALTH & FAMILY PLANNING

Hindus believe that a marriage can extend through a person's current incarnation to over seven lives. A husband and wife are considered linked by marriage both physically and spiritually, and sex outside marriage is strictly forbidden (although in practice, this ban is often less strictly enforced on men).

For most Hindus, there are no prescribed beliefs on birth control for married women, although it is frowned upon for unmarried couples, given the emphasis on marriage. However, both Hindu and Asian traditions stress the value of the family, children as the purpose of marriage, the sacred nature of conception, and the importance of motherhood in a woman's life. Accordingly, there is often strong social pressure on Hindu women to procreate.

Contraceptive methods that cause spotting or irregular periods may be unacceptable to a woman whose religious and household activities are restricted during menstruation; traditionally, Hindu women have been regarded as unclean during menstruation. Gynecological exams should also be avoided during this time, if possible.

Traditionally, fertility problems are attributed to the woman; men may refuse to undergo any fertility tests. In most cases, the husband prefers to be included in discussions of contraception or sterilization. In vitro fertilization is generally acceptable if both the egg and sperm come from the married couple; using donor cells may be problematic. However, some Hindus will reject it (notwithstanding the cultural pressure to produce children) because they see it as interfering with the natural order.

Because of the commandment to avoid harming any living thing, abortion has been traditionally condemned, but there is a great deal of variance on this issue within the religion. Many women will consider a termination in desperate situations, but confidentiality and emotional support are essential during these times. In cases where the mother's life is in danger, her health typically takes precedence over that of the unborn child. Even when abortion is deemed to be the right decision, patients may still believe that the bad karma from the violence lingers.

It is never acceptable to terminate a pregnancy because of an illness or deformity detected in the fetus, as this life is considered no less sacred than that of a healthy fetus (although this tenet notwithstanding, there are many such abortions in India each year). It may, however, be acceptable to some to selectively reduce the number of embryos that implant following a successful in vitro fertilization (IVF) treatment.

Some Hindus also feel that it is more acceptable to abort a female fetus, given the high value Indian society places on males, although this is uncommon in the United States.

PREGNANCY & BIRTH

Birth is an occasion for great celebration in many Hindu communities; it is especially exciting for the mother, as childbearing is thought to be one of a woman's duties.

Though there are many Hindu customs surrounding pregnancy and childbirth, they vary a great deal between families, communities, and geographical areas. For example, some mothers may wait to bathe after delivery until a religious bath can be performed; during this period, women will cleanse themselves with a sponge. Additionally, some mothers feel uncomfortable with their babies being bathed without their consent. Many mothers are also uncomfortable with their newborns being placed in a separate room, so communication is necessary between the patient and hospital staff if an infant must be moved into a nursery or NICU.

For some Hindus, a ceremony of welcome is performed for the baby, either at home or in the hospital. This ceremony includes writing "om," a sacred sound, on the baby's tongue with honey or ghee (clarified butter); because honey is not recommended for infants due to the risk of infant botulism, providers may need to discuss alternatives with parents. Hymns, mantras, and the name of God are whispered into the baby's ear. Some families may also wish to wrap the baby in a special cloth with religious significance. If a family chooses to perform this ceremony in the hospital, it is appreciated if privacy is given.

For some Hindus, a female close to the new mother symbolically washes the mother's breasts before she feeds her baby for the first time. Traditionally, the mother receives 40 days of rest after giving birth.

The mother may receive a large number of visitors, since birth is a cause for great celebration and extended family is generally expected to visit. Extra space in the room for visitors should be provided, if possible.

It may be important for some Hindu patients to know the exact time of birth so that they can get an accurate horoscope. The first letter of the baby's name may be chosen by the person who makes out the baby's horoscope. The full name is often chosen by an elder in the family or by a priest. This traditionally happens on the tenth day after birth.

Many traditional Hindus believe that the soul enters the body of the fetus during the seventh month of pregnancy. Thus, many families may wish to perform a proper religious funeral if a miscarriage occurs after this period. Before the seven-month mark is reached, whether religious rites are performed is commonly left to the discretion of the family. Some Hindus believe that miscarriage is the karmic fault of the mother; therefore, extra support may be necessary for the woman following a miscarriage or stillbirth.

In the case of stillbirth, the body should be wrapped in a towel or clean, white cloth and made available for the family to view.

END OF LIFE

Most Hindus prefer to die in their own homes, so death in the hospital may be very distressing for patient and family alike. If a terminal patient must remain in the hospital, staff should be prepared for a potentially large number of visitors; the space provided and visiting hours may require some adjustment.

The family should be consulted to see if they wish to perform the Last Rites in the hospital; a pundit (priest) may be brought in to administer them. Last Rites often include readings from the Bhagavad Gita or a holy text in a local language such as Gujarati or Tamil (for a non-US patient), tying of thread around the patient's wrist or neck, marking the forehead with blessed dust, sprinkling the patient with water from the Ganges, or placing a sacred tulsi leaf (basil) in the patient's mouth. Additionally, the family may bring money and clothes for the patient to touch so that they can be distributed to the needy in the patient's name after death.

Hindu tradition teaches that the body must return to nature. Thus, a dying patient may request to be placed on the ground during his/her final breaths to be closer to the earth.

The dying process requires a Hindu to concentrate his/her mind on a personal mantra, which creates the proper state of mind for an easy reincarnation. However, if the patient is unconscious, it is customary for a family member to chant a mantra in the person's right ear and to place holy ash on his/her forehead.

Some Hindu families are extremely concerned with who touches the body after death. If no family members are available, the following procedure should be observed:

- Do not remove sacred items like threads or jewelry from the body, and consult the family before touching the body. If it is necessary to remove these items, the use of gloves is appreciated.

- Close the patient's eyes, straighten his/her limbs, and wrap the body in a plain sheet.

- Do not cut nails or trim hair without the family's consent.

- In most cases, the body should not be washed, since this is part of the funeral rites and will usually be carried out by relatives at a later time.

- If a body must be left in a room overnight, a light or candle should be left to illuminate the room.

- If possible, the body should be placed with the head pointing north and the feet south.

- If the family requests a viewing of the body, staff should ensure that the room is free of any religious symbols.

Most Hindus will not allow a postmortem unless it is legally essential, since opening the body is believed to be disrespectful to the dead and his/her family. If it is necessary, the patient's family will most likely insist that all organs be returned to the body for cremation (all Hindus over age five are cremated).

If possible, less than 24 hours should pass before the funeral; the death certificate should be filled out as quickly as possible so that funeral arrangements can be carried out. Traditionally, in the death of an adult, the eldest son is responsible for making funeral arrangements. If the body remains at the hospital for more than a day, it is likely that extended family and friends will visit to pay their last respects, a binding duty for many Hindus.

Mourning rituals may last for over a year. There is a strong bond between the living and the dead, since many Hindus believe that dead family members help the deceased's spirit to progress through the worlds of ancestral spirits until the time of its next rebirth.

FOR MORE READING: HINDUISM

Ghadiali H. Hinduism and medicine. In: Goodacre D, ed. *World Religions and Medicine*. 2nd ed. Oxford, UK: Institute of Religion and Medicine. 1983: 15-23.

Knipe, DM. Hinduism and the tradition of Ayurveda. In: Sullivan LE, ed. *Healing and Restoring: Health and Medicine in the World's Religious Traditions*. New York, NY: Macmillan. 1989: 89-109.

Metropolitan Chicago Healthcare Council. (2004). Quick reference for health care providers interacting with Hindu patients and their families. Kentucky Hospital Association Web site. http://www.kyha.com/documents/QR-ALL.pdf. Published March 23, 2005. Accessed August 17, 2008.

Mysorekar U. Spirituality in palliative care: A Hindu perspective. In: Puchalski CM, ed. *A Time for Listening and Caring: Spirituality and the Care of the Chronically Ill and Dying*. Oxford, UK: Oxford University Press. 2006: 171-182.

Schott J, Henley A. Hinduism. In: Schott J, Henley A, eds. *Culture, Religion and Childbearing in a Multiracial Society*. Oxford, UK: Butterworth-Heinemann. 1996: 304-311.

PART 3: RELIGIONS OF THE WORLD & THEIR APPLICATIONS TO HEALTH CARE

6. Sikhism

Overview FAQ

1. When, where, and how did Sikhism originate?
Sikhism was founded in the 15th century in Northern India and Pakistan by Guru Nanak. The teachings of Guru Nanak and his nine successors, also called gurus, form the basis of the religion.

According to Sikh tradition, Guru Nanak went to the river to bathe and meditate one morning and remained there for three days. While meditating, he had an epiphany about the nature of God. When he returned to his village after the three days of meditation, he announced, "There is no Hindu and no Muslim," emphasizing the need for humans to transcend sectarian differences. He then began traveling the Indian and Arabian peninsulas, spreading his message of a single, omnipresent God and salvation through spiritual union with God.

Each of the ensuing nine gurus expanded on and reinforced the message of his predecessor. Their teachings became the foundation for the Sikh religion.

2. Does Sikhism have sacred texts? What are they called?
The primary sacred text of Sikhism is the *Guru Granth Sahib*.

The fifth Sikh Guru created an official version of the *Guru Granth Sahib* in 1604, with additional text added later by the 10th Guru. The text is comprised of nearly 6,000 hymns (*shabads*) and teaches its adherents how to live a life of peace, tranquility, and spiritual enlightenment. Sikhs recognize this text as a living, perpetual guru to guide all adherents.

3. What are the core beliefs of Sikhism?
The core belief in Sikhism is faith in *Vahiguru*, an infinite, formless, and eternal, creator. Sikhism also places an emphasis on absolute equality among humans, living life in an honest way, remembering God, and sharing with those in need.

Sikhism teaches that adherents must develop an intimate faith and relationship with *Vahiguru*. The goal is liberation, which is achieved not after death but while living in the world of activity. Human beings who are able to control and diminish their ego are able to realize *Vahiguru* and achieve liberation, provided this process is accompanied by grace. Before salvation is realized, humans' souls may be continuously reincarnated and unable to unify with *Vahiguru* due to the Five Vices: ego, anger, greed, attachment, and lust.

4. What are the core practices of Sikhism?

Initiated Sikhs wear five articles of faith at all times. These articles make up an external uniform that Sikhs use to identify themselves. The articles, all starting with the letter "k" (commonly called the "Five Ks") are:

1. **Kesh**: uncut hair on any part of the body, which is mandatory for both men and women; a turban (*Dastaar*) covers the uncut hair of men and some women;

2. **Kangha**: a small wooden comb for the maintenance of the uncut hair that symbolizes social commitment;

3. **Kara**: a steel bracelet that reminds Sikhs to engage in ethical conduct;

4. **Kachhera**: cotton underwear (resembling knee-length shorts) which reflect the dignity, modesty, and high moral character of the wearer; and

5. **Kirpan**: a sword that represents the duty to seek justice and fight oppression. While there is no prescribed length, *kirpans* are typically between 3 and 6 inches long.

The gurdwara ("doorway to divinity") is a Sikh house of worship and learning. *Gurdwaras* serve as community centers, teaching halls, meeting places, and the location for religious ceremonies. Each *gurdwara* has a kitchen (*langar*) where food is prepared and given freely to anyone, regardless of their faith.

5. What are Sikhism's important holidays? How are they celebrated?

For a Sikh, there are no holidays in the traditional sense. Every day is to be celebrated and should be used as an opportunity to become closer to God.

In practice, many Sikhs do gather in large numbers at local *gurdwaras* to observe certain days during the year. These gatherings typically mark a historically significant occasion, such as *Gurpurabs,* days that mark the birth or martyrdom of the Gurus. The *Gurpurabs* include:

- **Vaisakhi,** the day the tenth Guru, Guru Gobind Singh, created the *Khalsa Panth* (the order of initiated Sikhs) and formalized the Sikh identity

- The **birthday of Guru Nanak,** founder of Sikhism

- The **birthday of Guru Gobind Singh,** the 10th Guru

❧ The **martyrdom of Guru Arjan**, the fifth Guru

6. How many adherents of Sikhism are there in the United States? Are they located in a particular region?

There are approximately 500,000 Sikhs residing in the United States. Areas with large Sikh populations can be found all over the country, from Yuba City, California to Queens, New York, from Española, New Mexico to the state of Oregon, and large cities including Chicago, Seattle, Detroit, and Houston.

7. What are the main sects or denominations within Sikhism?

Sikhism is a relatively young tradition and has not faced theological issues that would cause serious divisions. Rather, in the Sikh community, there has always been a large mainstream community with minor groups periodically emerging and then disappearing.

• • • •

Intersections with Health Care: FAQ

1. Does Sikhism have a particular view about what causes illness? Are there illness-related rituals?

While Sikh patients may consider their illness to be the will of *Vahiguru* (God), the religion generally stresses that the individual must make an effort to get well because human life is considered sacred. During times of illness, many Sikhs pray to *Vahiguru* for their health.

Since Sikhism originated in South Asia, some Sikhs may choose to combine Western health care with traditional medicine, including homeopathy and herbal medication.

2. Does Sikhism prescribe a particular type of dress for men or women?

Central to Sikh practice is wearing the articles of faith (i.e., the Five Ks). All initiated men and women are required to wear their hair long and uncut (kesh), and to maintain a steel bracelet (kara), sword (kirpan), wooden comb (kangha), and long underpants (kachera). It is extremely important that none of the Five Ks are removed from a Sikh without consent. If it is necessary to remove any of them, it is important to store them in a respectful space (e.g., *not* on the floor or near anyone's feet).

If hair from any part of the body must be removed, discuss this with the patient in advance. If hair is cut from the head, it should be given back to the patient for his/her own disposal.

Additionally, most Sikh men cover their hair with a turban, while women wear a long scarf (a *chuni*) over their heads and shoulders.

Both men and women may cover their bodies as much as possible during examinations and remove clothing only when necessary. If a hospital gown is required, Sikh patients should be offered one that reaches the ankles and is not open in the back. Many will feel more comfortable if allowed to wear a shawl or dressing gown over the gown while remaining in possession of the Five Ks.

3. Are there any prayer or ritual observances that are likely to occur during the patient's stay?

Many Sikhs spend a significant amount of time in meditative contemplation; this may include prayer and recitation from a prayer book. Many worship early in the morning, in the evening, and again before sleep. Before each prayer, it is customary for Sikhs to wash their hands or body.

Some Sikhs will have a prayer book, containing devotional hymns in the hospital room. Health care providers should ask permission before touching it, and if it is granted, wear disposable gloves to handle it. The book should never be placed near feet, on the floor, or in any location that is unclean; if in doubt, speak with your patient about what this means for him/her.

Sikhs – both male and female – who wear a turban will want to remove and re-tie their turbans once a day; if they are unable to do so, assistance should be offered. The assistant should either wash his/her hands or wear disposable gloves when handling the turban.

Some Sikh patients may also wish to play devotional music during the day; if this disturbs other patients, offer headphones that do not interfere with the turban (e.g., small, in-ear headphones).

4. Does Sikhism have hygiene or washing requirements?

Cleanliness is extremely important in Sikhism. As mentioned above, many Sikhs cleanse themselves with running water before meditation. If running water is not available, the patient should be offered a bowl and jug of water.

If a Sikh patient is unable to wash, dry, or comb his/her hair, help should be offered as it is traditional for Sikhs to maintain a clean and dignified appearance at all times.

Sikhs do not cut their hair, and males do not shave their beards. If hair needs to be shaved or cut for medical purposes, approach the patient with great sensitivity and, if at all possible, discuss the need with the patient in advance. It is quite possible that a Sikh will refuse a medical procedure if it would require hair to be removed from their body – this decision is up to the individual's discretion. It is also important to limit the amount cut to the extent medically necessary.

5. Are there any dietary restrictions?

One of the four central taboos in Sikhism is a bar on eating meat that has been ritually slaughtered or prepared for another religion (e.g., kosher or halal meat). Some Sikhs will extend this rule to all meat and meat products, and even eggs, fish, and dairy products. Given the different stringency with which these rules are observed, each patient should be consulted. However, vegetarian food is always a safe option. Another of the four central taboos relates to the consumption of intoxicants, including alcohol and tobacco.

It is common for Sikhs to have friends and family who visit and bring food from the *langar* (the communal kitchen inside Sikh places of worship). Eating *langar* food can be very comforting and should be allowed unless there are medical restrictions.

6. Are there any medications, treatments, or procedures that Sikhs cannot accept?

Many Sikhs avoid consuming anything that they believe will cause either temporary or permanent damage to their bodies. This includes tobacco, alcohol, and all narcotic or intoxicating drugs. However, most Sikhs will take medication that contains traces of alcohol or narcotics as long as the intention is not intoxication; the individual patient should be consulted when this is required.

If a certain medication contains animal products then the patient should be consulted. Generally, if the Sikh patient is a vegetarian, it will be impermissible for him/her to take this medication, and alternative medication should be offered.

7. Can Sikh patients see providers of the opposite sex?

There are no religious rules or restrictions that prohibit Sikh patients from seeing providers of the opposite sex, even with OB/GYN physicians or staff. However, culturally, some Sikhs may feel inhibited when discussing various aspects of their health, especially sexual matters. If this is the case, patients should be seen by a provider of the same sex.

8. Can Sikhs donate organs or accept donor organs?

Receiving and giving organs is accepted by the majority of Sikhs; the tradition teaches that the body is a temporary vessel.

9. Should I consult anyone other than the patient when seeking informed consent or other patient decisions?

Generally, Sikh families expect to be involved with the health care decisions of relatives. Some Sikhs, particularly the elderly, may refuse treatment if the family has not given its consent. Providers should discuss this with patients and learn which family members should be consulted.

10. What is Sikhism's view on reproductive health and family planning? Are contraceptives okay? What about abortion? Voluntary sterilization?

There are no religious mandates on these issues, and they are open to individual interpretation. Therefore, the decision to use contraception or undergo an abortion/sterilization rests with the patient. However, most Sikhs are of South Asian descent, and in South Asian culture, most people would prefer not use contraception, sterilization, or have an abortion. Ultimately, it is essential to speak with each patient to assess their personal beliefs on topics such as these.

11. Are there particular beliefs or rituals concerning pregnancy and birth? What about postpartum women? What about women who have miscarried?

A Sikh mother may be uncomfortable if her child is removed from her hospital room to a nursery or NICU. If it is necessary to separate mother and child, the reasons should be clearly explained.

Sikh babies are often not given an official name until the family visits their *gurdwara* for a naming ceremony. Medical records will need to be updated after the ceremony.

If a Sikh woman miscarries, the fetal remains should be wrapped in a clean, white cloth and given to the family for burial or cremation in accordance with local laws. It is important that the health care provider *not* cut a lock of hair from the child, as this is strictly forbidden.

Although the Sikh religion does not place any restriction on leaving the home after giving birth, some Sikh women follow the cultural practice of not leaving their homes for 40 days. If a Sikh woman is following this cultural tradition, if possible, postnatal appointments should be conducted via home visit.

12. Are there important end-of-life rituals or beliefs?

Most Sikhs will be visited by a *granthi*, someone who has studied the Sikh scriptures extensively. This person might wish to read from the scripture, such as the *Guru Granth Sahib*, and pray with the patient.

It is customary for a large number of relatives and close friends to visit, since visiting the ill is a Sikh duty. If possible, provide a space to accommodate the visitors. Visitors may wish to place written hymns or prayers beside the patient. After a Sikh has passed away, loved ones may recite sacred hymns together.

Sikhism teaches that the soul has departed and the flesh is empty when neither the heartbeat nor breathing can be restored; most Sikhs accept brain death as the departure of the soul from the body, and believe that attempts at resuscitation should not be taken to extremes. Once there has been a determination of death, the empty flesh left behind is not considered sacred. However, the body should be treated with great respect out of deference to and support of the family.

13. What should be done with the body after death?

Health care providers who come into contact with the body should wear disposable gloves, cover any open wounds, close the eyes and mouth, and straighten the arms and legs. If possible, the body should *not* be washed, as this is believed to be the family's duty. Additionally, it is extremely important that the articles of faith not be removed, including any hair or a Sikh's turban. The body should be wrapped in a clean, white cloth. It is preferable that these procedures are done by a health care provider of the same sex as the patient.

Most Sikhs will not object to a postmortem.

• • • •

Sikhism: Intersections with Health Care

For its adherents, Sikhism is more a way of life than a set of religious tenets. One of its central ideals is that all life is to be preserved, so it tends to adapt easily to innovations in technology and health care that serve this end. Many Sikhs will gladly accept technological advances such as procedures for infertility treatment, organ donation, and genetic engineering—although many will reject procedures that they believe go against the principle of preservation of life, such as terminating a pregnancy.

Quick answers for many questions that arise when caring for a Sikh patient may be found in the FAQ. For more in-depth explanations, consult the appropriate section below.

CAUSES OF ILLNESS & HEALING RITUALS

As mentioned above, Sikhism teaches that protecting human life is a religious requirement; human life is viewed as a gift from the divine and is the highest form of all life. Many Sikhs believe that when life ends, the soul returns to the divine and that illness is the will of *Vahiguru* (God). However, there is a fine balance struck between the will of *Vahiguru* to give and take life, and the responsibility to preserve one's own health. Generally, individual Sikhs accept that the state of one's health is ultimately in the hands of *Vahiguru*, but that it is the individual's religious duty to do whatever s/he can to preserve the sanctity of his/her own life.

When illness strikes, Sikhs pray to *Vahiguru* for help, either alone or with trusted friends and family. Some also recite from the Sikh scripture, the *Guru Granth Sahib*, which is believed to provide physical and spiritual strength and nourishment. Some Sikh patients may ask that devotional music (called *kirtan*) be played.

Because Sikhism originated in South Asia, some Sikhs may choose to combine Western health care with alternative medicine, including homeopathy, naturopathy, and herbal medications. Some also rely on Ayurveda, a medical system developed on the Indian subcontinent that relies on the medicinal properties of natural substances (herbs, minerals, metals, fruits and vegetables, and animals) and on the physiological effects of certain foods and flavors.

INFORMED CONSENT & PATIENT DECISION MAKING

Given the importance Sikhism places on providing care for relatives, many Sikhs will expect their families to be involved in health care decisions. Some Sikhs, particularly the elderly, may refuse treatment if the family has not given its consent. Most Sikhs, regardless of age, will feel more comfortable making a decision with family input. Thus, it is usually important for the health care provider to involve the family.

GENDER & MODESTY

There are no religious rules or restrictions that prohibit Sikh patients from seeing providers of the opposite sex, even with OB/GYN physicians or staff. However, culturally, some Sikhs may feel inhibited when discussing various aspects of their health, especially sexual matters. If this is the case, patients should be seen by a provider of the same sex. If a facility cannot accommodate this, younger Sikhs, both male and female, may feel more comfortable if accompanied by a family member. However, this is strictly a matter of modesty rather than a religious teaching.

DRESS & MODESTY

Initiated Sikhs (called Khalsa Sikhs) wear five articles of faith, at all times. They also serve as an external uniform that Sikhs use to identify themselves. Young children and even infants may wear one or more of the Five Ks.

The articles, all starting with the letter "k" (commonly called the "Five Ks") are:

1. **Kesh**: uncut hair on any part of the body, which is mandatory for both men and women; a turban (*Dastaar*) covers the uncut hair of men and some women;

2. **Kangha**: a small wooden comb for the maintenance of the uncut hair and that symbolizes social commitment;

3. **Kara**: a steel bracelet that reminds Sikhs to engage in ethical conduct ;

4. **Kachhera**: cotton underwear (resembling knee-length shorts) which reflect the dignity, modesty, and high moral character of the wearer; and

5. **Kirpan**: a sword that represents the duty to seek justice and fight oppression. While there is no prescribed length, *kirpans* are typically between 3 and 6 inches long.

Most Sikh patients will want to retain these items on their persons as long as possible. If *any* of the articles are removed without patient consent, the patient may well feel as though s/he has been severely insulted and that his/her religious identity has been stripped away. Thus, it is extremely important that patient consent be sought any time a health care provider wants or needs to remove—or even handle—one of these items. Before removing or handling the Five Ks, it is also important to discuss how the articles of faith will be treated once removed.

Staff should reassure the patient that the items will be handled with the greatest respect. The articles should be placed only in a respectful space (e.g., not on the floor, near anyone's feet, or tossed in a bag with the patient's dirty laundry or other possessions).

The first article of faith, kesh (uncut hair), may prove an extra challenge for health care providers. Many Sikhs believe that keeping one's hair long and uncut confirms belief in the acceptance of divine will. Thus, if hair must be removed from any part of the body for a medical procedure, the patient should be advised as far in advance as possible so s/he can decide whether to proceed, and if so, get accustomed to the idea.

If hair must be removed, there are ways to try and reduce the trauma. Most importantly, providers should remove the minimum amount that is medically necessary for a given procedure. When hair is removed from the head, it should be given back to the patient for disposal. If hair must be removed from the body, there is also a specific prohibition against razors and scissors; should a patient adamantly reject the use of these implements, a depilatory cream might be an acceptable compromise.

Other than the articles of faith and their associated requirements, Sikh dress varies enormously – there are no actual guidelines requiring a particular style of dress or garment. Traditional dress is long, loose trousers and a long-sleeved jacket for men, and a pair of long trousers and overdress for women (called a *salwar-kameez*). Many

Sikhs in the United States—especially younger adherents—wear Western-style clothing.

Additionally, many Sikh men and some Sikh women cover their hair with a turban. Women who do not wear a turban might wear a long scarf (called a *chuni*) over their heads and shoulders. If these need to be removed, patients should be offered another head covering, if possible. As a religious observance, many men re-tie their turbans every day. If assistance is needed, the provider should either wash his/her hands or put on disposable gloves before touching the turban.

Although there is no specified dress, there is still a concern for modesty. Both men and women may choose to cover their bodies as much as possible during examinations and remove clothing only if needed. If a hospital gown is necessary, Sikh patients should be offered one that reaches the ankles and is not open in the back; many will feel more comfortable if they're allowed to wear a shawl or dressing gown.

PRAYER & RITUAL OBSERVANCES

Sikhs spend a significant amount of time in meditative contemplation; prayer and meditation are the cornerstones of Sikhism and the main practices that Sikhs employ in striving to become closer to *Vahiguru*. Sikhs customarily pray three times during the day—in the morning, early evening, and before bed. If possible staff should avoid interrupting these prayers for routine matters (e.g., taking a patient's blood pressure or temperature). Staff can ask patients about their prayer practices and the time of day they pray upon admission and schedule routine testing accordingly.

Although prayer is a highly individualized ritual, there are some aspects of its practice with which patients may require assistance. For example, many Sikhs wash before prayer. Running water is preferred, but patients with limited mobility may use a bowl of water. For some prayers, a Sikh may choose to stand while praying. Again, those with limited mobility may require some assistance or modifications to their normal routine.

Meditative time includes prayer and recitation from a prayer book that contains devotional hymns from the Sikh scripture, the *Guru Granth Sahib*. Sikhs are likely to have a copy of the text with them in the hospital, and it is considered insulting if the text is not handled with proper respect. Providers should ask permission before touching the text, and, if permission is granted, wear disposable gloves. The book should never be placed near feet, on the floor, or in any unclean location.

Sikh patients may also play tapes of devotional music (*kirtan*) during the day. This music comprises of songs from the *Guru Granth Sahib*; every verse of the text has an accompanying melody. Listening to *kirtan* is likely to comfort the patient. However, if it disturbs others, the patient should be offered a pair of headphones that do not interfere with his/her head scarf or turban.

It may be difficult for a Sikh patient who is hospitalized for an extended period of time to be separated from his/her community. One of the guidelines for living a disciplined Sikh life (along with prayer and meditation) is taking an active role in the safety and well-being of the community and of others generally. Many Sikhs volunteer in their local *gurdwara* or community center, or do other community service work not specifically related to their *gurdwara*.

During a prolonged hospital stay, it may become important to help the patient maintain his/her connection to the larger community. The patient's community will most likely help this process along by performing another Sikh duty - visiting the sick and bringing food from the *langar* (the *gurdwara*'s kitchen). Some of this food may be high in fat or sugar, requiring a conversation with the patient and family if the patient has hospital-imposed dietary restrictions.

HYGIENE & WASHING REQUIREMENTS

Sikhism teaches that physical cleanliness is necessary for spiritual cleanliness. The second article of faith, the *kangha* (comb), signifies the importance of keeping oneself physically and spiritually uncontaminated. Most Sikhs prefer to use running water for washing.

In addition to wearing the *kangha*, Sikhs maintain their hygiene through frequent cleansing with running water; many hospitalized Sikh patients will want to take a shower or bath every day. If the patient's health does not allow him/her to take a bath or use a sink, s/he should be offered a bowl and jug of water. Many Sikhs also wash their faces and hands before prayer or meditation, after eating, and after using the toilet. Before meditation, patients may also wish to change into clean clothes, if clothing has been soiled.

Given that uncut hair, *kesh*, is an article of faith and that Sikhism emphasizes cleanliness, Sikhs will wish to wash (with shampoo and conditioner) and dry their hair on a regular basis; at a minimum, most will want to brush their hair daily. Many Sikh men will treat facial hair the same way. Hair may be left to dry naturally, but if the patient prefers an electric hairdryer, assistance should be offered. After washing or brushing, the Sikh will need to re-tie his/her turban, for which he/she may also require assistance.

DIETARY REQUIREMENTS

One of the four founding taboos in Sikhism is not to eat any meat that has been ritually slaughtered (e.g., kosher or halal meats). The prohibition on kosher meat stems from a larger belief that all food is pure and does not require priestly inspection or intervention; the prohibition on halal meat comes from the commandment that only meat from animals killed quickly with a single blow (*jhakta* meat) is acceptable. Since halal requires allowing the blood to drain slowly from the animal, animals killed in this way are unacceptable.

However, while the *Guru Granth Sahib* seems to indicate that the prohibition on meat extends *only* to meat that has been ritually prepared for another tradition, there are wide variations in how individual adherents interpret this text. Some Sikhs will extend this rule to cover all meat and meat products, and even eggs, fish, and dairy; others will eat any meat as long as it is *jhakta* and is not beef or pork. Given the different stringency with which this prohibition is interpreted and observed, each patient should be consulted as to his/her individual practices.

Friends and family may also bring hospitalized patients food from the *langar* of the local *gurdwara*. This food, which is given freely to those in need, is always vegetarian so that people of any caste, culture, tradition, or religious background can consume it. *Langar* food is often a good option, as it both allows patients to maintain links to their communities *and* to continue eating their usual foods. However, if *langar* food is not a feasible option (either because the patient is on a medically restricted diet or because of a hospital policy against outside food), and the patient's views on eating meat are not clear, vegetarian food is always a safe option.

In addition to prohibitions around certain foods, Sikhism also prohibits consumption of anything that is believed to do either temporary or permanent damage to one's body. In Sikhism, the ultimate goal is to discover the divine spark within one's self. Because the physical body is the container for this divinity, Sikhs are enjoined from harming their bodies. Prohibitions are specifically enumerated in the *Guru Granth Sahib* and include tobacco, alcohol, and all narcotic or intoxicating drugs.

MEDICATION, TREATMENT, OR PROCEDURE RESTRICTIONS

In general, there are no religious prohibitions on any medications in Sikhism; most Sikhs will even take medication that contains alcohol or narcotics as long as the intention is to heal, and not to become intoxicated.

Leniency is less likely to be given for medication that does not meet Sikh dietary requirements. Many Sikhs practice vegetarianism and will not want to accept medication that contains animal byproducts; as a general rule, vegetarian medication should be offered if it is available. If there are no treatment options that meet Sikh dietary requirements, this should be clearly explained and discussed with the patient.

REPRODUCTIVE HEATH AND FAMILY PLANNING

When Sikhs marry, it is believed that the two individual souls of the spouses become spiritually united. Thus, marriage is thought of as a semi-holy state and elevates the partners' spiritual states; as such, it is strongly encouraged.

Most Sikhs, particularly those from older generations, discourage all sexual relations outside of marriage, believing that it is immoral.

Sikhism also teaches that lust (*kam*) is one of the five major vices and that sexual activity should be restricted to sex between married partners. When an unmarried Sikh seeks medical attention for an issue related to sexual activity, s/he may be uncomfortable and will appreciate extra sensitivity, especially if the patient is a minor or is accompanied by family members who may be unaware of his/her sexual activity. Hysterectomies must be discussed with extra care. Many Sikh women are from South Asian backgrounds. They are likely to feel that they are failing to meet a cultural standard, and may also face family pressure against the procedure. If a hysterectomy is medically inevitable, counseling (either religious or secular) may be required to help the patient come to terms with her medical condition, and it may be important to involve her spouse. As, most Sikhs are of South Asian descent, and in South Asian culture, most people would prefer not use contraception, sterilization, or have an abortion it is ultimately essential to speak with each patient to assess their personal beliefs on topics such as these.

PREGNANCY & BIRTH

Birth is an occasion for great celebration in the Sikh tradition, as new children are seen as the cultural wealth of a family and the consummation of a married couple's spiritual union. New parents are likely to receive a large number of visitors. Relatives may bring a bracelet (*kara*) for the infant, which should not be removed without parental consent.

Observant Sikh women giving birth will most likely want to remain in possession of all Five Ks. Unless this poses a health threat, it should be allowed. Some very devout Sikh women will not want to remove their *kachera* (underwear), even during birth. If it becomes an obstacle to care and the provider seeks its removal, women may choose to leave one leg or an ankle in the *kachera* as a compromise.

Sikh mothers very rarely let their new children out of their sight; thus, many will be uncomfortable if the baby is removed from the mother's room to a nursery or NICU. If this practice is necessary in a particular facility, the health care provider should take time to explain to the mother the reason behind the removal.

Although the Sikh religion has no rule about leaving the home after giving birth, some Sikh women follow the cultural practice of not leaving their homes for 40 days after giving birth. If a Sikh woman is following this cultural tradition, if possible, postnatal appointments should be conducted via home visit. During this period, female relatives and members of the faith community visit frequently to ensure that all the mother's and household's needs are being met.

Once the mother and child are able to travel, the family usually visits their *gurdwara* for a naming ceremony and celebration of the birth. During this ceremony, the *Guru Granth Sahib* is opened to a random page. The first letter of the first word on the left-hand page is used as the first letter of the child's name. If the baby is a boy, *Singh* (meaning "lion") will also be added as a surname; for a baby girl, *Kaur* (meaning "princess") will be added. Once the official name is chosen, medical records will need to be updated.

If a woman miscarries, the child's body (or the birth products, depending on the stage of pregnancy when the miscarriage occurred) should be wrapped in a clean cloth and given to the family for proper washing, burial, or cremation, in accordance with local law. Washing in particular is seen as the family's duty. In addition, providers should not cut a lock of hair from the child, as it is religiously forbidden to cut hair even at this early stage.

ORGAN DONATION

Organ donation is generally permissible in Sikhism, based on two religious beliefs.

First, Sikhism teaches that saving a human life is one of the greatest things a person can do. Second, Sikhism teaches that while the soul is eternal, the body is only its perishable shell and is no longer sacred once the spark of life is gone. Thus, if another person can be helped through use of the "shell," organ donation is a positive act.

Personal objections or discomfort with organ donations may override these religious principles, however, so each patient and his/her family should be consulted.

END OF LIFE

It is customary for a large number of relatives and close friends to visit if death is imminent, because visiting the ill is a Sikh duty. Family will expect to be closely involved in end-of-life treatment and decisions, although the patient retains the final say. If the hospital staff is overwhelmed by a large number of visitors, the facility may ask the family to designate one or two close relatives who are allowed to visit, especially in sensitive hospital areas like the ICU. Relatives may also be asked to limit the number visiting and then rotate and take turns.

Most severely ill Sikhs will be visited by a *granthi*, a person who has studied the Sikh scripture extensively. The *granthi* will read from the scripture and pray with the patient to spiritually prepare him/her for death. Visitors may wish to place written hymns or prayers beside the patient.

As in most religions, the topic of when it is one's divinely determined time for death versus the obligation to provide medical intervention to prolong life is a very sensitive one. For Sikhs, there are two sets of competing interests.

First, there is the Sikh belief that human life is a gift from *Vahiguru*. Sikhism teaches that one who does not appreciate this gift will have to face direct consequences. Second, although it is generally taught that every effort must be made to preserve life, Sikhs believe that the dying adherent has an opportunity to reunite with *Vahiguru*. Thus, preserving life in a vegetative state may be seen as unnecessarily keeping the patient separated from the divine.

As a result, discussions regarding the termination of life support, Do Not Resuscitate orders or whether or not to pursue extraordinary measures are likely to be sensitive. If a patient or family is struggling with these difficult issues, it is wise to bring in the counsel of a Sikh religious leader or chaplain, who can respond to the questions and concerns of the patient.

Sikhism teaches that the soul has departed and the flesh is empty when neither the heartbeat nor breathing can be restored; most Sikhs accept brain death as the departure of the soul from the body, and believe that attempts at resuscitation should not be taken to extremes. Once there has been a determination of death, the empty flesh left behind is not considered sacred. However, the body should be treated with great respect out of deference to and support of the family.

All health care staff should wear disposable gloves when touching the body; if possible, the person handling the body should be of the same sex as the deceased. All open wounds should be covered, the eyes and mouth closed, and the arms and legs straightened. The body should not be undressed, and should be wrapped in a clean, white cloth. It is extremely important that the articles of faith not be removed, including any hair from the patient or a male Sikh's turban.

Cleansing the body is a religious ritual for Sikhs; many families will wish to do this themselves and feel very uncomfortable if the body is washed by hospital staff. The family might ask to prepare the body in the hospital, and facilities should be made available if possible. If this cannot be accommodated, the reasons why should be clearly explained to the deceased's family and attempts at compromise made.

Most Sikhs will not object to a postmortem, if it is recommended.

FOR MORE READING: SIKHISM

Ethnicity Online (2003). Cultural Awareness in Healthcare: Sikhs. Ethnicity Online web site http://www.ethnicityonline.net/sikh.htm. Accessed November 12, 2008.

North American Sikh Medical and Dental Association (2000) Sikhism News. http://www.sikhdocs.org sikhism-news/index.php. Accessed Thursday, December 04, 2008.

Schott J, Henley A. Sikhism. In: Schott J, Henley A, eds. *Culture, Religion and Childbearing in a Multiracial Society*. Oxford, UK: Butterworth-Heinemann. 1996: 343-348.

Sikh Coalition (2001). About Sikhism: Resources.
Sikh Coalition Website http://www.sikhcoalition.org/InfoEducators.asp.
Accessed November 21, 2008.

Sikh Women (2000). Sikh Patient's Protocol for Health Care Providers. Guidelines for Healthcare Providers Interacting with Patients of the Sikh Religion and Their Families. Sikh Women Website. http://www.sikhwomen.org
Accessed December 1, 2008.

7. Shintō

• • • •

Overview FAQ

1. When, where, and how did Shintō originate?
Shintō is indigenous to Japan, and its start can be traced to ancient Japanese religions and to the origin of Japan itself. Its origins are considered to date back to the era before an organized Japan was established, making it impossible to identify with precision when Shintō came to exist.

Basic elements of modern Shintō can be traced to 300 BCE–250 AD. Shintō was the official Japanese state religion from the 19th century through the end of World War II.

It is important to note that many practitioners identify with more than one tradition: someone may be both Shintō and Buddhist.

2. Does Shintō have sacred texts? What are they called?
Though Shintō does not have official scripture, there are texts with "privileged" status, including the *Kojiki* (Records of Ancient Matters) and the *Nihon-gi* (Chronicles of Japan). They were written in 712 and 720 and are the compilations of ancient Shintō oral traditions, mythology, and ceremonies. In Shintō, one will not find written texts of religious precepts or commandments.

3. What are Shintō's core beliefs?
Shintō centers on the worship of *kami* ("that which is hidden") or spirits; different kami are venerated to bring about different effects. Every living and nonliving thing is believed to contain a kami; they are the sacred or mystical element in everything. Shintō teaches that there are an infinite number of kami. While everything is believed to contain kami, only creatures or objects exhibiting it in a striking way are referred to and/or worshiped as such. The most worshipped kami is *Amaterasu*, the Sun Goddess.

4. What are Shintō's core practices?
The most important Shintō practice is the worship of kami at shrines. This is done most often at public shrines, although it is also common for Shintō to have small shrines in their homes. Purification rites are also important; Shintō rituals and personal practices aim to cleanse both the body and the mind. Both water and salt are commonly used in purification rites, and it is common to see Shintō cleanse their faces, mouths, and hands with pure water before worship.

Shintō also observes various *matsuri* (festivals) throughout the year (see below).

5. What are Shintō's important holidays? How are they celebrated?

Shintō festivals center on the kami who is the guest of honor for the occasion. The festivals celebrated by a Shintō depend on which kami s/he worships. The festivals are often very bright, colorful, and loud, and feature a feast and sometimes sumo wrestling.

The most attended festival and most important holiday of the year occurs on January 1, the Japanese New Year (*Oshogatsu*). On this day, people go to a shrine to thank the kami and to ask for good fortune for the coming year. Also widely celebrated is *Kinensai*, a spring festival dedicated to praying for a good rice harvest.

November 23 is *Kinrokansha-no-hi*. Now a national holiday honoring labor, it was originally a Shintō Harvest festival where the Emperor dedicated the year's new rice to the gods; this observance is still practiced in the Imperial Household.

Additionally, there are annual festivals (*Rei-Sai*) held on the important dates particular to each public shrine. On these days, ceremonies take place within the shrine, while the local kami are carried in effigy around the town, accompanied by music and dancers.

6. How many Shintō are there in the United States? Are they located in a particular region?

An estimated 60,000 Taoists and Shintō reside in the United States. However, because Shintō is so closely tied to the Japanese way of life and so many Shintō also observe another religion, it is difficult to pinpoint an exact number.

7. What are the main sects or denominations within Shintōism?

Scholars divide Shintō into four types: Folk, Sect, Shrine, and State.

- **Folk Shintō** practices include spirit possession, shamanic healing, and divination, mostly derived from local, ancient traditions.

- **Sect Shintō** is comprised of 13 groups formed during the 19th century. Sect Shintō does not have shrines, but conducts worship in meeting halls.

- **Shrine Shintō** is the oldest and most prevalent sect, and is said to have existed throughout all of Japanese history. An organization called *Jinjya-Honcho* maintains the shrines and works to uphold the fundamental principles of Shintō.

- **State Shintō** refers to the practice of Shintō that occurred from the 19th century through World War II. During this period, Shintō was the official state religion of Japan, and Buddhist and Confucian ideals were shunned. Following World War II, State Shintō was abolished.

PART 3: RELIGIONS OF THE WORLD & THEIR APPLICATIONS TO HEALTH CARE

••••
Intersections with Health Care: FAQ

1. Does Shintō have a particular view about what causes illness? Are there illness-related rituals?

Shintō is based on the worship of kami, which are spirits/spiritual essences inhabiting every living and non-living thing (kami means "that which is hidden").

There are a vast number of kami associated with healing, both for specific ailments and for healing in general. For example, *Mekura-gami* and *Idono-Kami* are kami for illness of eyes, while *Tsuri Tenjin* is the kami of stomach illnesses. The list of illness-related kami is quite extensive, and which kami are worshiped during times of illness is left to the individual decision of the patient.

Patients who are able to travel may choose to visit the shrine of the kami affiliated with the particular type of healing they require. At the shrine, the individual may perform *ohyakudo*, in which the practitioner walks around shrine 100 times (or as many times as their age or health status allows). These pilgrimages are believed to aid the healing process, sometimes causing miraculous recoveries.

While most Shintō utilize Western medicine, some use a medical system called *Kampō* that dates back to sixth-century Japan. Kampō diagnoses are based on the combined number of symptoms a patient exhibits, which the Kampō doctor detects through auditory, tactile, olfactory, and visual tests. Treatment of nearly any ailment usually consists of acupuncture and herbal medicine.

2. Does Shintō prescribe a particular type of dress for men or women?

Almost all Shintō wear clothes particular to their culture, not their religion.

In Japan, amulets and charms from shrines and temples are very popular. The amulets and charms are inscribed with the name of their temples of origin and purpose (e.g., health maintenance, good luck, prosperity). They can be worn on the person (e.g., as a pendant) or attached to something else; in Japan, it is a popular practice to hang an amulet from the hospital bed. They should not be removed without patient consent.

3. Are there any prayer or ritual observances that are likely to occur during the patient's stay?

Some Shintō patients may set up a shrine in their rooms called a *kami-dana* (kami shelf); it is customary to place flowers and fresh food and water at the shrine each morning. The kami shelf often contains a tiny replica of a traditional Shintō shrine, a mirror, and amulets. Visitors, especially family, may bring religious objects to place on the shelf, and prayers may be performed in front of it. The shrine, or any objects on it, should not be touched without patient consent.

4. Does Shintō have hygiene or washing requirements?

Many Shintō follow Japanese cleansing rituals and practices such as washing the hands, face, and mouth with pure water prior to worship. Water may also be sprinkled outside an entranceway to purify the area, and baths are taken before bed so as not to dirty the mattress.

In Japan, nightly bathing is often discontinued when one becomes ill and is resumed only after a doctor gives permission. Thus, patients might ask their doctors when they can bathe at night again; when the doctor grants permission it is seen as a sign of recovery. Visitors may choose to bring gifts that symbolize purification and cleanliness, such as soap and cologne.

5. Are there any dietary restrictions?

Most Shintō eat a traditional Japanese diet; Shintō does not have any specific dietary prescriptions. The Japanese diet largely consists of fish, steamed vegetables, fresh fruit, rice, and herbal teas.

6. Are there any medications, treatments, or procedures that Shintō cannot accept?

Western medicine is the most popular form of health care for most Shintō in the United States; there are unlikely to be any objections to any medications, treatments, or procedures.

7. Can Shintō patients see providers of the opposite sex?

Shintō are generally reserved and value privacy, and may wish to have their own rooms. The value placed on privacy does not necessarily translate into the need to see a provider of the same sex; however, each patient should be consulted.

8. Can a Shintō donate organs or accept donor organs?

Shintō are permitted to both donate and receive organs.

9. Should I consult anyone other than the patient when seeking informed consent or other patient decisions?

Many Shintō follow the Japanese practice of joint decision making, wherein important decisions are made after a reasonable agreement is reached among concerned individuals. In the case of health care decisions, this will often mean the patient and his/her family, particularly elders.

It is also traditional for a doctor to give any grave prognoses to the most important family members first. This may become an issue for providers, especially in cases where there is a language barrier and providers are relying on family members to translate.

10. What are Shintō's views on reproductive health and family planning? Are contraceptives okay? What about abortion? Voluntary sterilization?

Birth control is used heavily in Japan, and the vast majority of Shintō have no objection to the use of contraceptives.

Shintō defines life as starting at birth, so abortions are generally more accepted within this tradition than they may be in other religions; they are often accepted as a necessary evil. Stances on abortion are much more likely to reflect the Japanese attitude, which is largely one of acceptance, than religious beliefs.

Often, abortions and miscarriages are followed by ceremonies or memorial services.

11. Are there particular beliefs or rituals concerning pregnancy and birth? What about postpartum women?

Birth is seen as a moment of great joy and celebration, and there are many commemorative ceremonies that attend it. Most Shintō women prefer to give birth in a hospital, not at home. Many will want close relatives to be in the room, although not involved in the actual delivery.

Traditionally in Japan, new mothers stayed at home for three weeks following birth, although contemporary Japanese tend not to follow this practice.

12. Are there end-of-life rituals or beliefs I need to know about?

There are no formal rituals for end-of-life care in Shintō. Shintō teaches that death and the dead are impure, making it inappropriate for Shintō priests to deal with them. Despite this belief, a Shintō patient will likely be surrounded by many loved ones as death approaches.

Because priests do not deal with the dead, there are no funerary rites and virtually no Shintō cemeteries. However, because the majority of people that practice Shintō have beliefs that are amenable to other religions (especially Buddhism), family members often carry out either cultural death rites or the death rituals of another religion.

13. What should be done with the body after death?

Shintō does not prescribe specific treatment for a dead body; the patient's family will make these decisions.

• • • •

Shintō: Intersections with Health Care

Shintō is an ancient Japanese religious tradition with a wealth of beliefs and practices around health and illness and a variety of healing rituals. Visits to shrines and herbal remedies are often employed; there is a panoply of shrines and deities believed to provide relief for almost any illness or symptom.

In addition to traditional healing methods, Shintō has a unique outlook on end-of-life issues: it regards death and dying as unclean and inappropriate for Shintō to deal with, and has no end-of-life rituals or funerary rites.

Quick answers for many questions that arise when caring for a Shintō patient may be found in the FAQ. For more in-depth explanations, consult the appropriate section below.

CAUSES OF ILLNESS & HEALING RITUALS

Shintō is based on the worship of kami, which are spirits/spiritual essences inhabiting every living and non-living thing (kami means "that which is hidden"). Shintō teaches that there are an infinite number of kami. While everything is believed to contain kami, only those exhibiting it in a striking way are referred to and/or worshipped as such. The most worshipped kami is Amaterasu, the Sun Goddess.

There are a vast number of kami associated with healing, both for specific ailments and for healing in general. For example, Mekura-gami is a kami for illness of eyes, while Tsuri Tenjin is the kami of stomach illnesses. The list of illness-related kami is quite extensive, and which kami are worshiped during times of illness is left to the individual decision of the patient.

Patients who are able to travel may choose to visit the shrine of the kami affiliated with the particular type of healing they require. At the shrine, the individual may perform ohyakudo, a ritual in which the individual walks around the shrine 100 times or as many times as their age or health status allows (there are also shortened versions of this ceremony). These pilgrimages are believed to aid the healing process, sometimes causing miraculous recoveries.

The most popular pilgrimage destination is the Ishikiri Shrine, just outside Osaka, Japan. Many Japanese visit this shrine in time of illness to perform ohyakodu; patients who have visited the shrine may have amulets. Other shrines with particular curative properties—of which there are hundreds—may also be visited. For example, there are shrines believed to aid in childbirth, shrines for the general health of children, shrines for resolving ear infections, and more.

Despite the popularity of worship and pilgrimage as healing methods, Western medicine is the most popular form of health care for most Shintō, and there are unlikely to be any objections to any medications, treatments, procedures, or organ donation.

Some practitioners may also choose to use a medical system called Kampō that dates back to seventh-century Japan, which is not Shintō-specific but is widely used in Japan. Kampō diagnoses are based on the combined number of symptoms that a patient experiences, which the Kampō doctor detects through auditory, tactile, olfactory, and visual tests.

Treatment of nearly any ailment consists of acupuncture, moxibustion (a traditional healing technique based on burning the herb mugwort), and herbal medicine. The combination of treatments used is determined by the gender, age, and constitution of the patient, in addition to the climate in which the patient resides. Diagnoses are highly individual, but herbal treatments for each diagnosis are fixed according to prescriptions in classical Chinese texts (where Kampō originated before being exported to Japan).

Kampō coexists with Western medicine for most Shintō; in Japan, some Kampō treatments are covered by the national health insurance program and many pharmacies have staff trained in prescribing herbal remedies. In addition, in the United States, several Kampō herbal remedies are currently in clinical trials. Kampō treatment may be offered by acupuncturists, naturopaths, and other alternative medicine practitioners.

DRESS & MODESTY

Almost all Shintō wear clothes particular to their culture, not their religion. Shintō priests wear a garment called a *jo-e*, made from white or yellow silk, along with a peaked cap (*tate-eboshi*), an outer robe that looks like a kimono (*jo-e no sode-gukuri no o*), an undergarment (*hitoe*), a girdle (*jo-e no ate-obi*), and a pair of trousers. However, it is unlikely that one would see this outfit within a health care setting, since this clothing is worn by priests only during religious ceremonies.

In Japan, amulets and charms from shrines and temples are very popular. The amulets and charms are inscribed with the name of their temples or shrines of origin and purpose (e.g., health maintenance, good luck, prosperity); they are sold at stands surrounding the temples. They can be worn on the person (e.g., as a pendant) or attached to something else; in Japan, patients sometimes hang amulets from their hospital bed, although they are most often kept in handbags or wallets. They should not be removed without patient consent.

HYGIENE & WASHING REQUIREMENTS

Shintō has a strong emphasis on maintaining cleanliness and purity, including physical purity; being unclean is viewed as an insult to the gods. Thus, for most Shintō, cleanliness is extremely important. In their own homes, most will remove their footwear and will bathe, wash their hands, and rinse out their mouths frequently.

Before worship, most Shintō wash their hands and mouth with pure water. To accommodate this, the patient should be provided with access to running water or, in the case of limited-mobility patients, a jug of water and a bowl. Water may also be sprinkled outside an entranceway to purify the area, and baths are taken before bed so as not to dirty the mattress.

In Japan, nightly bathing is often discontinued when one becomes ill and is resumed only after a doctor gives permission. Thus, patients might ask their doctors when they can bathe at night again; when the doctor grants permission, it is seen as a sign of recovery. Visitors may choose to bring gifts that symbolize purification and cleanliness, such as soap.

PRAYER & RITUAL OBSERVANCES

Worship at a shrine is central to Shintō life, and Shintō patients may choose to set up a shrine in their rooms, called a kami-dana (kami shelf); each morning, it is customary to place special items at the shrine including plants (ideally, a Japanese *Sakaki* tree, a small evergreen plant that is the sacred tree of Shintō), fresh food (e.g., rice), and/or water. The shrine is often a shelf that contains a tiny replica of the sanctuary of a shrine, a mirror, and amulets.

Adherents will pray at the shrine, either to ask a kami for help or to thank a kami for its assistance. Shintō worship typically has four components:

1. *Purification.* Prayer is usually preceded by ritual cleansing, which involves washing the hands and mouth (see Hygiene & Washing Requirements). Salt is sometimes also used for purification; providers should be aware of this if treating a Shintō patient on a low-sodium diet;

2. An *offering*, such as some grains of rice or a cup of sake (Japanese rice wine);

3. *Prayer*; and

4. *Feasting*.

However, at a home or hospital-room shrine, worship can be as simple as pausing to bow in front of the shrine.

Visitors, especially family, may choose to bring religious objects to place on a home or hospital-room shrine, and may pray for the assistance of kami. The shrine or any objects on it should not be touched without patient consent, and should be handled carefully, if at all.

DIETARY REQUIREMENTS
Most Shintō eat a traditional Japanese diet; Shintō does not have any specific dietary prescriptions. The Japanese diet largely consists of fish, steamed vegetables, fresh fruit, rice, and herbal teas.

MEDICATION, TREATMENT, OR PROCEDURE RESTRICTIONS
Western medicine is the most popular form of health care for most Shintō in the United States; there are unlikely to be any objections to any medications, treatments, or procedures.

GENDER & MODESTY
Shintō are generally reserved and value privacy and may wish to have their own rooms when possible. The value placed on privacy does not necessarily translate into the need to see a provider of the same sex; however, each patient should be consulted for his/her preferences.

Culturally, the patient may also be more reserved than most Western patients; this can be the case regardless of the genders of practitioner and patient. This reserve reflects the Shintō teaching that hierarchy is to be respected; thus, quietness on the patient's part typically indicates deference to the health care provider, not inattention or lack of concern.

INFORMED CONSENT & DECISION MAKING
Many Shintō follow the Japanese practice of joint decision making, wherein important decisions are made after a reasonable agreement is reached among concerned individuals. In the case of health care decisions, this will often mean the patient and his/her family, particularly elders.

Conversations around terminal prognoses and advance directives may be particularly difficult. Shintō does not deal with death or dying, seeing it as impure (see Hygiene & Washing Requirements and End of Life), so patients may not want to have these discussions. Elderly patients may defer to their children for these decisions.

It is also traditional for a doctor to give any grave prognoses to the most important family members first. They often keep it from the patient, believing that such a prognosis would be so difficult for the patient to cope with that it would hasten death. This may become an issue for providers, especially in cases where there is a language barrier and providers are relying on family members to translate.

REPRODUCTIVE HEALTH & FAMILY PLANNING
Birth control is used heavily in Japan and Shintō defines life as starting at birth, so that the vast majority of Shintō have no objection to the use of contraceptives.

Although they may be frowned upon, abortions are more accepted within Shintō than in some other religious traditions. Generally, Shintō teaches that abortion is an affront to the kami who provided the seed for the fetus; however, it is often accepted as a necessary evil. Any moral objection is lessened by the belief that life begins at birth.

Whether an adherent of Shintō opposes abortion or not is more often based on cultural rather than religious ties. For example, in Japan, abortion is much more accepted than in other nations, reflected in their extremely low birthrate.

Despite widespread acceptance, abortion is never taken lightly. Often, abortions are followed by ceremonies or memorial services (particularly, *mizuko kuyo*, or water ceremonies). Mizuko kuyo are services that are held once a month in which those that have lost a child (whether through abortion, miscarriage, stillbirth, or during infancy) gather in the morning at a temple, pay a fee, and have their names recorded on small wooden tablets. Those in attendance then participate in an hour-long service, during which parts of the Lotus Sutra (a Buddhist scripture which has been assimilated into Shintō) are chanted; this is accompanied by beating drums and a talk by a priest, if one is present. This is normally followed by an informal hour of socializing at the temple. It is important to note that these ceremonies take place at temples, not shrines; temples are the appropriate location for everyday ritual and practice, while shrines are places of worship and celebration for special events.

PREGNANCY & BIRTH

Birth is seen as a moment of great joy and celebration, and there are many commemorative ceremonies that attend it. The most important and common ceremony is the introduction of the child to the kami in his/her community. In Japan, it is customary for mothers to take their babies to the shrines in their communities to introduce the child to the kami for protection.

Most Shintō women prefer to give birth in a hospital, not at home. Many will want close relatives to be in the room, although not involved in the actual delivery.

Traditionally in Japan, new mothers stay at home for three weeks following birth, although contemporary Japanese tend not to follow this practice.

Following a stillbirth or early infant death, parents may want to hold a memorial service (see Reproductive Health & Family Planning).

ORGAN DONATION

Shintō scholars are split as to whether or not organ donation is permissible. The fraction that supports organ transplantation from brain-dead donors do so on the grounds that offering an organ to a recipient whose life is dependent upon it is a community service, something highly valued in the Shintō tradition. However, before the recipient receives the organ, a ritual is often performed in which the soul of the donor is first transferred to the spiritual world. This ritual can only be conducted when the person is considered deceased under Shintō requirements (see End of Life).[9]

The majority of Shintō scholars, however, oppose all organ transplantation from brain-dead donors, even if the ritual of spiritual transference has been performed. Shintō teaches that the soul of the deceased maintains a special relationship (called *itai*) with descendents. Many believe that organ transplantation injures this relationship between ancestors and their kin.

In addition, Shintō teaches that being natural and pure are among the highest priorities; organ donation is viewed as unnatural and therefore undesirable. Additionally,

---

[9] The ritual for organ donation is not based on Shintō thought. It is determined by the person who hopes to have the ritual.

there is a concern that the potential recipient might wish for the expedient death of the donor, which is a harmful way of thinking.

Physicians seeking permission for organ donation from a Shintō family must approach them with extreme sensitivity. If the family is willing to allow donation, providers should facilitate the soul-transference ceremony to ensure that the family is comfortable with the process.

END OF LIFE

A common saying in Japan is that "one lives as a Shintō and dies as a Buddhist." Because of Shintō's emphasis on purity and cleanliness, terminal illness, dying, and death are considered impure and inappropriate for Shintō priests to deal with. There are virtually no Shintō cemeteries or end-of-life rituals, and candid discussions about a patient's prognosis may be difficult. Older patients may wish to leave the decision making to their children; given the high value placed on reserve in both Shintō and Japanese culture generally, privacy for these difficult conversations would be appreciated.

Despite the belief in the impurity of death, Shintō is extremely family-oriented and a Shintō patient will likely be surrounded by many loved ones as death approaches. What should be done with the body after death should be a decision made by the patient and his/her family.

The actual moment of death according to Shintō tradition is not easily translated into Western medical practice; some Shintō will not accept brain-death as death, making conversations about organ donation even trickier. Shintō teaches that an individual is only temporarily dead when his/her soul leaves the body (e.g., there is no sign of brain activity); permanent death must be religiously confirmed.

In some regions of Japan, a ritual called *tamayobai* is performed, in which close relatives or friends shout out the name of the deceased immediately after his/her heart stops beating. This is done with hopes that a spiritual miracle might revive the person. Thus, it is important to confirm with the family that a Shintō patient is deceased before any post death practices are performed.

Since the majority of people that practice Shintō have beliefs that are amenable to other religions, the individual and/or family members will often wish to carry out either cultural death rites or the death rituals of another religion. These will most commonly be Buddhist rituals (unless the patient had converted to another religion during life), as the Japanese view Buddhism as the religious tradition that deals with death.

FOR MORE READING: SHINTŌ

Kobayashi K, Okabe T, et al. People of Japanese descent. In: Waxler-Morrison N, Anderson JM, Richardson E, and Chambers NA. *Cross-Cultural Caring: A Handbook for Health Professionals*. 2nd ed. Vancouver, BC: UBC Press. 2005: 163-196.

Leininger M. Japanese Americans and culture care. In: Leininger M, McFarland MR, eds. *Transcultural Nursing: Concepts, Theories, Research and Practice*. 3rd ed. New York, NY: McGraw-Hill. 2002: 453-464.

Ohnuki-Tierney E. Health care in contemporary Japanese religions. In: *Healing and Restoring: Health and Medicine in the World's Religious Traditions*. Sullivan LE, ed. New York, NY: Macmillan. 1989: 59-87.

Spector RE. *Health and Illness in the Asian Population*. Upper Saddle River, NJ: Pearson Education. 2004: 209-229.

8. Traditional Chinese

Taoism, Confucianism, and Chinese Folk Religion: Overview FAQ

1. When, where, and how did Chinese religions originate?
Three main religious traditions can trace their origins to China: Chinese folk religion, Confucianism, and Taoism. They all evolved from ancient East Asian cultures and developed into unique belief systems. Many practitioners identify with more than one tradition: someone may practice both Chinese folk religion and Confucianism.

- **Chinese folk religion** is not based on particular founders, creeds, theologies, or organizations. Rather, it is a series of beliefs and rituals that have been transmitted from generation to generation by the Chinese people. As such, it dates back thousands of years to ancient Chinese spiritual practices and does not have a single date of origin.

- **Confucianism** developed from the teachings of the Chinese sage and philosopher Confucius (551–479 BCE). Though his teachings were not accepted during his lifetime, Confucianism was adopted as China's State Philosophy and the code of ethics for the Chinese people in the first century BCE. Note that while many Chinese value Confucian virtues and strive to practice them, it is uncommon for someone to self-identify as "Confucian."

- **Taoism** has evolved throughout Chinese history. While its roots can be traced to prehistoric Chinese religions, many consider the origin of its philosophy to be the composition of the *Tao Te Ching* in the late fourth-early third century BCE, while the religion formally developed in the second century BCE.

In addition to these three Chinese belief systems, it is also important to note that Buddhism has also long been practiced in China. For more information, see the Buddhism chapter.

2. Do Chinese religions have sacred texts? What are they called?

- **Chinese folk religion** has no official sacred texts, although some believers view Confucian and Taoist texts as sacred.

- **Confucianism's** sacred texts are the *Five Classics* and *Four Books*. The first volume of the Four Books is the *Lun Yu* (Analects of Confucius). It is the most revered Confucian text and contains his principal teachings as compiled by the second generation of his followers.
  The other three volumes are the *Chung Yung* (Doctrine of the Mean), *Ta Hsueh* (Great Learning), and *Meng Tzu* (Mencius). In addition, Confucian tradition teaches that there are Five Classics that were revered by Confucius: *Shu Ching* (Classic of History), *Shih Ching* (Classic of Odes), *I Ching* (Classic of Changes), *Ch'un Chiu* (Spring and Autumn Annals), and *Li Chi* (Classic of Rites).

- The most important **Taoist** text is the *Tao Te Ching* (The Way and Its Power). Its origins are debated; some contend that it was written by Lao Tzu during the sixth century, while others believe that it was written by anonymous authors over several centuries. Most Taoists consider the Tao Te Ching to be the essential guide to living a full spiritual and ethical life.
  There are also additional Taoist texts on which different sects choose to focus. These are often revealed transmissions from perfected beings, saints, and avatars who now live in higher realms and reveal the secret workings of the cosmos.

3. What are the core beliefs of Chinese religions?

- **Chinese folk religion** is largely *animistic* (i.e., it teaches that objects found in nature, like trees, rivers, rocks, and mountains have souls). Ancestors may also be considered sacred, as may famous cultural heroes, either from myth or history; on occasion, nature deities are also revered. The religion is based on the assumption that the spirit world influences the course of human events.
  The natural phenomena are understood as the product of the cosmological forces of *yin* (dark, feminine) and *yang* (light, masculine). When yin and yang are balanced, there will be harmony, manifested in social and familial stability and prosperity. Also necessary for balance are proper relationships between the earth and the *ch'i* (immanent powers); heaven and the *shen* (spirits); and humanity and the *kuei* (ghosts).

- **Confucianism** teaches that humans must try to align their behavior with the *Tao* ("the way of nature"). Like Chinese folk traditions, Confucianism also believes in the forces of yin and yang, and teaches that the tension between yin and yang results in an endless process of change, which is the natural order. The goal of practitioners is to flow with this process and align their behavior and society as a whole with the natural order.

Confucianism also emphasizes the importance of relationships and of sympathizing with others, especially during times of suffering. For many Confucians, the highest virtue is *Ren*, or benevolence toward others. Confucianism teaches that in order to achieve the ultimate personal and social harmony in life, one must maintain the five proper relationships: ruler to subject, parent to child, husband to wife, older to younger, and friend to friend.

- **Taoists** have a hierarchy of deities, which include gods and goddesses, immortal humans, and ancestors. There are also deities for every occasion and element of nature. Presiding over the entire pantheon are *San Ch'ing* ("The Three Pure Ones"), the highest deities.

  The concept of Tao is arguably the most important belief in Taoism. However, it is believed that Tao cannot be described in words. Tao is the ultimate, inexpressible, indefinable source of creation that gives rise to all beings and influences the natural order. Taoist theology focuses on the doctrine of non-action (*wu-wei*), the goal of which is a state of perfect accord with the Tao, or *p'u* (simplicity).

4. What are the core practices of Chinese religions?

- **Chinese folk religion** is often characterized as ritualistic—emphasizing proper external devotion over internal worship. Through offering incense, paper talismans, or food, practitioners draw the gods near to ward off negative influences, ask for future blessings, or give thanks for blessings received. Before rituals, it is common for believers to dress in clean clothing or to alter their diet or fast to enter a state of moral correctness and ritual purity.

- It is difficult to codify the core practices of **Confucianism** because it is primarily an ethical system whose practices vary depending on the believer. However, it is often argued that the central purpose behind Confucian practices is to uphold harmony in the "Five Relationships": ruler to subject, parent to child, husband to wife, older to younger, and friend to friend. For example, a parent owes a child education, care, and moral guidance, while a child owes a parent obedience, respect, and care in old age. Though obedience and deference are demanded from subordinates in all five relationships, harmonious relationships are viewed as mutually beneficial.

- True understanding of **Taoist** practice can only be obtained through study with a Taoist master because many of the religion's practical elements are taught through an oral tradition. However, there are some practices that are common and well-known. Recitation of the Tao Te Ching is an important spiritual practice for many Taoists. Reciting the words is believed to have the power to banish evil spirits, bring good luck, prolong life, and cure sickness. Meditation is a prominent practice, and it is thought to give the believer mental space to know the Tao directly. Controlled breathing is also an important practice, as it is the most easily observed form of the flow of energy in the universe.

5. What are the Chinese religions' important holidays? How are they celebrated?

- The most important holiday celebrated in **Chinese folk religion** is the New Year. The Chinese New Year is celebrated over a period of two weeks at the beginning of the Chinese lunar year (which falls in late January-early February). Celebration includes rituals, which may include the worship of Heaven and Earth, worship of gods important to the family, and veneration of ancestors. At the conclusion of these rites, it is common to hold a family feast to reaffirm the family's unity. The celebration ends with a lantern festival, in which people hang glowing lanterns in temples and carry them in an evening parade. Additionally, it is customary to wear red, as that color symbolizes fire and is believed to drive away bad luck.

- Two important holidays for **Confucianism** are Confucius Day and the Chinese New Year (see above). The former celebrates the birth of Confucius and has been celebrated for thousands of years. On this day, Confucian ritualists perform commemorative rituals in temples or halls following a strict 37-step ceremonial sequence, including elaborate dances and a memorial service. In China, Confucius Day coincides with National Teacher's Day in honor of Confucius' pedagogical contributions to civilization.

- The most widely celebrated holiday in **Taoism** is the Chinese New Year (see above). Taoists celebrate the Three Pure Ones with an offering of sweets, an exchange of gifts, and a feast. On the first day of the festival, there is a Dragon/Lion Dance, which celebrates immortality and union with the spirits. There are other festivals throughout the year which celebrate the birth of deities and the solstices. Of particular importance is the celebration of Lao Tzu's birthday on the 15th day of the second lunar month; it is considered to be the most important Taoist holy day.

6. How many adherents of Chinese religions are there in the United States? Are they located in a particular region?

There are an estimated 3.6 million Chinese Americans, however, it is unknown how many practice Chinese religions. Additionally, there is no estimate for how many non-Chinese Americans practice these religions. The cities with the largest Chinese American populations are Boston, New York City, San Francisco, Los Angeles, Washington, DC, and Houston.

7. What are the main sects or denominations within Chinese religions?

- Though **Chinese folk religion** and **Confucianism** are extremely diverse, there are no formal divisions within these traditions.

- **Taoism** has no central organization or hierarchy, which makes naming sects within the tradition tenuous. Some divide Northern Taoism (practiced in mainland China) from Southern Taoism (practiced in Taiwan and South China). Others divide the religion into three different organizations: literati, communal, and self-cultivation. Literati Taoists are often members of the educated elite who focus on Taoist ideals expressed by ancient thinkers' classical texts. Communal Taoists include members from all levels of society and have priestly hierarchies and regular rituals. Self-cultivation Taoists focus on personal well-being, peace of mind, and spiritual immortality. However, none of these divisions are rigid.

• • • •

Intersections with Health Care: FAQ

1. Do these religious traditions have a particular view about what causes illness? Are there illness-related rituals?

Traditionally, Chinese medicine teaches that health is a state of spiritual and physical harmony with nature. For Confucians, harmony is disrupted if someone fails to observe the five basic relationships of society. In Taoism, harmony results from a proper balance between humans and nature. In all three traditions, a disruption of this harmony can manifest itself in illness.

Taoism and Confucianism also teach that the body is composed of five solid organs (*ts'ang*, the liver, heart, spleen, lungs, and kidneys) and five hollow organs (*fu*, the gallbladder, stomach, large intestine, small intestine, and bladder). These organs have a complex relationship that helps maintain harmony within the body.

Illness-related issues should be discussed with great sensitivity. According to Chinese tradition, discussing problems and negative events aloud can bring bad luck.

2. Do these religious traditions prescribe a particular type of dress for men or women?

Patients may have amulets that protect their health and ward off evil spirits. Amulets usually contain a charm painted with an idol or Chinese characters. Amulets may be worn in the hair, pinned on clothing, hung over a door, or hung on a wall. Jade is also thought to have a positive correlation with health and patients may wear jade charms.

Neither the amulets nor jade charms should be removed without the patient's consent. If consent is given, they should be treated with extra care.

3. Are there any prayer, ceremonial, or health-related rituals that are likely to occur during the patient's stay?

Healing practices are highly ritualized, often involving clergy who preside over the manipulation of written texts. Rituals may also include water, plants, tree species, swords, seals, talismans, and mirrors.

Traditional Chinese medicine employs acupuncture, in which the body is punctured with special needles by a trained practitioner. The needles are inserted into 365 points on the skin. By inserting needles into the proper points, the acupuncturist can unblock the flow of *q'i* (the vital energy that gives life to all living matter), which restores health. Given the strong Chinese influence in Taoism and Confucianism, patients of these religions may also choose acupuncture treatment.

Traditional Chinese medicine also uses *moxibustion* to restore the balance; it is believed to be particularly useful during labor and delivery. In moxibustion, a properly trained healer heats pulverized wormwood and applies it directly to the skin on certain key points.

Another Chinese traditional healing practice called *cupping* may also be performed. The practitioner burns the oxygen out of a small glass (thus creating a vacuum) and applies the glass it to the patient's skin. This is believed to increase circulation and is often done to treat lung congestion. Cupping may leave bruise-like marks on the patient's body.

Medicinal herbs are also important in Chinese medicine. The most widely used is ginseng, which is believed to stimulate digestion, work as a sedative, help faintness after childbirth, and restore health to frail children. It is used in many forms, including powder, in broth or a brew, or raw. If a provider believes that the herbs will interfere with a patient's Western medical treatment, communication between the patient and provider is essential.

4. Do these religious traditions have hygiene or washing requirements?

No, Chinese folk religion, Confucianism, and Taoism do not prescribe particular hygiene or washing requirements. Adherents will most likely follow the cultural customs.

5. Are there any dietary restrictions?

Diet is more likely to be based on culture rather than religion. However, those following a strictly religious diet will balance foods that are *hot* and *cold*. Whether a food is considered hot or cold is not based on temperature, but on type. For example, most fruit and vegetables are cold, while red meat and spices are hot. Certain ailments may require avoiding one or the other type of food.

6. Are there any medications, treatments, or procedures that adherents of these traditions cannot accept?

For cultural reasons, practitioners of Chinese religions may resist having blood drawn and, because of its unfamiliarity, traditional Chinese physicians do not use blood samples in diagnosis, but rely on external evaluation.

Health care providers may not know when a patient is unsatisfied with a particular practice or situation; some patients of Asian backgrounds may choose to remain stoic and not voice complaints. This does not necessarily mean that nothing is wrong, but providers may need to ask more questions to ensure that the patient is satisfied.

7. Can patients from these traditions see providers of the opposite sex?

Many patients will not resist seeing a provider of the opposite sex; however, each should be asked for their preference.

8. Can adherents of these traditions donate organs or accept donor organs?

Given the resistance to drawing blood and the reluctance to have intrusive surgical procedures, there may be a cultural objection to organ donation and reception. The patient should be asked for his/her preferences.

9. Should I consult anyone other than the patient when seeking informed consent or other patient decisions?

Patients that practice Taoism, Confucianism, and Chinese folk medicine are likely to have strong bonds with their families. For many, maintaining the hierarchy of their family structures will be extremely important. Thus, family elders will often be involved in decision making.

10. What are these religious traditions' views on reproductive health and family planning? Are contraceptives okay? What about abortion? Voluntary sterilization?

Family planning decisions are often made on cultural, not religious grounds. Contraceptives are allowed; the most common form of birth control in China is the intrauterine device. Oral contraceptives are available at no cost to Chinese citizens and sterilization is common.

There are a range of religious beliefs in Confucianism, Taoism, and Chinese folk religion on abortion. However, these are often overridden by its cultural acceptability.

11. Are there particular beliefs or rituals concerning pregnancy and birth? What about postpartum women? What about women who have miscarried?

There are a variety of folk beliefs around pregnancy. Some Chinese women believe that talking about their pregnancy in the first trimester may attract bad luck. The expectant mother's diet is also thought to be very important in ensuring a healthy pregnancy. Pregnancy, particularly the second and third trimesters, is traditionally regarded as a hot condition, and expectant mothers may cut back on those foods (see Dietary Requirements). After birth, a mother is considered to be in a cold condition, and therefore might cover herself with extra clothing and eat hot foods; cold foods to avoid during this period include salads, cold drinks, steamed food, green vegetables, and ice cream.

In Chinese tradition, postnatal women are also encouraged to rest for the month after giving birth. In China, a mother typically stays in the hospital for five to seven days after delivery; reasons for a shorter stay may need to be explained to the family. Women may also use traditional Chinese medicines to encourage postbirth recovery.

Some mothers may be reluctant to bathe their children until the umbilical cord stumps have fallen off, fearing infection. Infants of Asian origin might develop harmless patches of bluish skin known as Mongolian spots; those unfamiliar with them may assume the spots are bruises.

In traditional Chinese culture, men are not present during labor or birth; the women are attended to by their mothers or other married female relatives. Since some believe that laboring women are particularly susceptible to sickness, they may prefer to have the windows closed at all times. Some families may wish to take the placenta home to bury it; each family should be asked for its preference.

Those practicing Taoism and Confucianism often believe in astrology, which is also an important part of Chinese traditional belief. For those for whom astrology is important, it is necessary to know the exact time of birth so that the child's horoscope is accurate.

In case of miscarriage, stillbirth, or neonatal death, most parents are unlikely to have any objection to a health care provider washing and wrapping the baby's body. However, each family should be asked for its preference.

12. Are there end-of-life rituals or beliefs I need to know about?

Death rituals vary considerably depending on culture.

In traditional Chinese culture, there are five funeral stages. Taoist or Confucian priests will likely be called to assist in these stages, depending on the religion of the deceased:

1. In the first stage, the dying person sees every member of his/her family before dying. This is a **familial obligation**, and the patient should be provided with a private room to accommodate the potentially large number of visitors if possible.

2. The second stage is **announcement** of the death to the community.

3. The third stage is **bathing** the body with fresh water so that the deceased can pass into the next world comfortably; providers should ask ahead of time to determine whether or not the body should be washed in the hospital.

4. The fourth stage is called **"the Lamp to Light the Way,"** in which family members place a plant-oil lamp at the feet of the corpse as mourners gather.

5. The fifth stage is **burial**. Traditionally, the deceased is not buried until resting in his/her house for three days.

Confucius did not believe in life after death. However, his *Book of Rites* contains strict rules for post death rituals and explains in great detail how the body should be arranged, how mourners should behave, what mourners should wear, and more.

In contrast to Confucianism, Taoism teaches that the deceased can become supernatural if s/he cultivates his/her moral character during life. Taoist funerary rites have four main components: chanting scriptures and litanies, water and land rituals, the lighting and disposal of lanterns, and the feeding of hungry ghosts. The extravagance of these ceremonies is dependent on the family's wealth.

13. What should be done with the body after death?
Many Chinese and Chinese Americans mix elements from multiple religions into funeral rites. Thus, each family should be asked for their preference on how to handle the body.

• • • •

Taoism, Confucianism, and Chinese Folk Religion: Intersections with Health Care

Religion in China is a complex, multifacted landscape, with a variety of overlapping religious traditions, including Buddhism, Taoism, Christianity, ancestor worship, and folk religion; many Chinese combine elements of two or more of China's religious traditions. In addition, China is home to a number of rich cultural and philosophical traditions, like Confucianism, that also meld with its religious tapestry. Belief systems based on the philosophical traditions of China have spread beyond the nation and are manifested throughout Asia.

Although there is a tremendous amount of diversity, there are some broad concepts shared across traditions, which exert a strong influence on how patients will understand health and illness. First, most traditional Chinese belief systems are not monotheistic, instead seeing the divine in nature, relationships between people, and the spirit world. Second, many have an emphasis on balance and harmony, both within the individual and between the natural and spirit worlds.

Quick answers for many questions that arise when caring for a Taoist, Confucian, or followers of Chinese folk religion may be found in the FAQ. For more in depth explanations, consult the appropriate section below.

CAUSES OF ILLNESS & HEALING RITUALS
Traditionally, Chinese medicine has taught that health is a state of spiritual and physical harmony with nature.

For Confucians, harmony is disrupted if someone fails to observe the five basic relationships of society, which are understood to be reciprocal relationships:

1. Ruler to subject;

2. Parent to child;

3. Husband to wife;

4. Older to younger; and

5. Friend to friend.

In Taoism, harmony is a result of the proper balance between humans and nature. Disruption is also thought to occur when there is an improper balance between yin and yang. Yin and yang are cosmic forces that are believed to animate all of nature. They are interdependent, complementary forces that can only exist in relation to one another.

In both the Confucian and the Taoist traditions, the disruption of harmony often manifests itself through illness. The inside of the body and its front are considered yin, while its surface and back are yang. Thus, yin is believed to store the vital strength of life, while yang protects the body from outside forces. If either the yin or the yang is out of balance, the other is put at risk.

In addition to the forces of yin and yang, Taoism and Confucianism teach that the body is composed of five solid organs (called ts'ang: the liver, heart, spleen, lungs, and kidneys) and five hollow organs (called fu: the gallbladder, stomach, large intestine, small intestine, and bladder). It is believed that the organs have a complex relationship that maintains harmony within the body; parts of the body that are considered yin must work in tandem with those considered yang in order for an individual to be healthy.

Taoism also teaches that illness and health do not occur only on the individual level, but also on the cosmic, universal level. One's health is not just dependent on harmony within the body, but is related to one's harmony with his/her ancestors, one's community, and with natural forces. Yin and yang dictate the harmony of all life; thus, for a proper balance of yin and yang, a sick individual must look beyond his/her individual body to seek balance in the surrounding world.

Traditional Chinese religion has many of its own healing practices, many of which have spread to the other Asian religious traditions:

- Chinese folk medicine employs acupuncture, an ancient practice in which the body is punctured with special needles by a trained practitioner. By inserting needles into the proper points, the acupuncturist can unblock the flow of q'i (the vital energy that gives life to all living matter), which restores health. Q'i is thought to run through the body along different channels, which a practitioner can access at 365 different points on the skin.

- Moxibustion is another traditional method of healing used to restore the proper balance of yin and yang; it is customarily done when it is believed that there is an excess of yin and is believed to be particularly useful during labor and delivery. In moxibustion, a properly trained healer heats pulverized wormwood (also called mugwort) and applies it directly to the skin on certain key points.

- A healing practice called cupping may also be performed. Cupping draws blood and lymph to the surface by burning the oxygen out of a small glass (thus creating a vacuum) and applying it to the person's skin. This is believed to increase circulation and is often done to treat lung congestion. Cupping may leave bruise-like marks on the patient's body that are sometimes mistaken for signs of abuse, especially in children.

Medicinal herbs are also important resources used by traditional Chinese healers. The most well-known herb used is ginseng, which is believed to stimulate digestion, work as a sedative, address faintness after childbirth, and restore health to frail children. It is used in a variety of ways: it can be rubbed on as a powder, prepared in broth or tea, or eaten raw. There are many other particular herbs and plants used for specific ailments that a patient may have. For providers to assess whether the use of herbs will interfere with a patient's Western medical treatment, communication between the patient and provider is essential.

PRAYER & RITUAL OBSERVANCES

In both Taoism and Confucianism, healing practices are highly ritualized and most often involve clergy presiding over manipulation of written texts. This may take the form of ritualized movements of either a writing brush or sword; this is believed to create harmony between the mind and body. Rituals may also include purification with water.

Patients of all three traditions may also have amulets to both protect their health and ward off evil spirits, a typical Chinese cultural practice. The amulets typically contain a charm with an idol or Chinese character painted in red or black ink on yellow paper. These amulets may be worn in the hair, pinned on clothing, hung over a door, placed on a wall, or placed inside of a red bag, as red symbolizes good luck, courage, loyalty, and honor. Jade is also positively correlated with good health, and Chinese patients may wear jade jewelry.

Neither the amulets nor jade charms should be removed without patient consent. If consent is given, they should be handled with respect; the jade charms should be treated with extra care. Some believe that if the jade is broken, they will be met with misfortune.

DRESS & MODESTY

Patients who do not wear Western clothing will most likely dress in accordance with their cultural backgrounds; Taoism, Confucianism, and Chinese folk religion have no traditions requiring specific types of dress.

GENDER & MODESTY

Most patients will not resist seeing a provider of the opposite sex. However, each patient should be asked for his/her preference. There are no religiously imposed restrictions or guidelines.

HYGIENE & WASHING REQUIREMENTS

Chinese folk religion, Confucianism, and Taoism prescribe no particular hygiene or washing requirements. Adherents will most likely follow their cultural customs.

DIETARY REQUIREMENTS

Diet is more likely to be based on culture rather than religion. However, those following a strictly religious diet will balance foods that are considered to be hot and cold. Yin food is considered "hot" while yang food is "cold". Whether a food is considered hot or cold is not based on temperature, but on type. For example, most fruit and vegetables are cold, while red meat and spices are hot. Additionally, boiled and steamed foods may be considered cold, while fried foods are hot.

How balance is achieved varies according to the health of the individual. For example, it is believed that a woman is prone to coldness postpartum. Thus, cold foods like fruits and vegetables are generally avoided. Because the list for yin versus yang foods is vast, the health care provider should discuss diet carefully with the patient.

Milk and dairy products are typically not consumed by most Chinese except those in the northern part of the country; the rate of lactose intolerance among Asians is higher than that of many other populations.

Rice is a staple of nearly every meal in Chinese cooking. Peanuts, soybeans, tofu, fried rice noodles, and pork are also popular in the Chinese diet. It is common for relatives to bring these foods to the patient; this should be allowed, if possible, as it will likely bring great comfort to the patient. However, health care providers should be aware that Chinese food often has a high sodium content. If this endangers the patient's health, the reasons for barring these foods should be explained.

MEDICATION, PROCEDURE, OR TREATMENT RESTRICTIONS

Those who practice Chinese religions may resist having blood drawn due to unfamiliarity stemming from the lack of this practice in traditional Chinese medicine (however, drawing blood was and is common as a result of some forms of acupuncture). Traditional Chinese physicians do not take blood to make a diagnosis, but rather examine the patient externally. This may also make some reluctant to have intrusive surgical procedures (anything that requires cutting into the body). However, this is more often a cultural rather than religious decision. If blood tests or surgical procedures are necessary, providers should be sure to clearly explain why and what it will entail.

INFORMED CONSENT & DECISION MAKING

Patients practicing Taoism, Confucianism, and Chinese folk religion are likely to have strong bonds with their families. For many, maintaining the hierarchy of their family structures will be extremely important. Thus, patients will often want the elders of the family to be involved in decision making.

The main exception to this practice is regarding issues of sexual health. Traditionally, sexual health, contraception, and contraceptives are not discussed openly (although this does not mean that they are not being used).

Regardless of who is involved in the decision making process, matters of health and illness should be discussed with great sensitivity. According to Chinese tradition, discussing problems and negative events aloud can bring bad luck. The health care provider should aim to present information in positive terms rather than negative (e.g., discuss the positive effects of a treatment in order to prevent negative effects of the illness rather than centering a conversation on the negative aspects of the illness or a negative prognosis).

Because of an Asian cultural emphasis on stoicism, health care providers may not know when a patient is unsatisfied with a particular treatment or resolution; patients may choose not to voice complaints. This does not necessarily mean that nothing is wrong, so providers may need to delve more deeply.

REPRODUCTIVE HEALTH & FAMILY PLANNING

Reproductive health and family planning decisions are most often made on cultural, not religious grounds. The most common form of birth control in China is the intrauterine device. Oral contraceptives are available at no cost to Chinese citizens and sterilization is common.

There are a range of religious beliefs in Confucianism, Taoism, and Chinese folk religion on abortion, which are usually secondary to cultural or political norms. Neither Taoist nor Confucian ethical codes explicitly forbid abortion, although it is generally viewed as a necessary evil to be chosen only as a last resort. However, because there are no strict religious rules outlawing it, patients have the option to decide for themselves whether or not it is ethical.

PREGNANCY & BIRTH

There are a variety of Chinese folk beliefs surrounding pregnancy.

Some traditional Chinese women believe that talking about their pregnancy in their first trimester may attract bad luck.

The expectant mother's diet is also thought to be very important in ensuring a healthy pregnancy. Pregnancy, particularly during the second and third trimester, is traditionally regarded as yang (a hot condition). Thus, those who eat a traditional diet may cut down on yang foods (e.g., red meat and fried foods). After birth, a mother is considered to be in yin (a cold condition) and therefore might cover herself with extra clothing and eat foods considered yang (hot) for at least a month. Foods to avoid during this period include salads, cold drinks, steamed food, green vegetables, and ice cream.

During labor, some Chinese women may be concerned about their vulnerability to illness caused by climate (e.g., wind, cold air) or ghosts, and may prefer to have all windows closed to lessen the possibility of sickness.

In Chinese tradition, postnatal women are encouraged to rest for the month after giving birth. In China, the mother traditionally stays in the hospital for five to seven days after delivery; if a shorter stay for normal births is typical in a particular facility, this may need to be explained to the family. Some women may also wish to use Chinese herbal medicines to encourage postbirth recovery or may choose to bathe themselves with a sponge for the month following birth.

Some mothers may be reluctant to bathe their children until the umbilical cord stumps have fallen off, fearing infection. Infants of Asian origin often develop harmless patches of bluish skin known as Mongolian spots; they are congenital birthmarks, but those unfamiliar with them may assume the spots are bruises.

In traditional Chinese culture, men are not present during labor or birth. Rather, the women are attended to by their mothers or other married female relatives. Some families may wish to take the placenta home to bury it; each family should be asked for its preference.

Practitioners of Taoism and Confucianism follow a wide range of beliefs in astrology, which is an important component of Chinese traditional belief. For those for whom astrology is important, it is necessary to know the exact time of birth so that the child's horoscope can be accurately prepared.

In case of miscarriage, stillbirth, or neonatal death, most parents are unlikely to have any objection to the health care provider washing and wrapping the baby's body. However, each family should be asked for its preference.

ORGAN DONATION

Given the resistance to drawing blood and the reluctance to have intrusive surgical procedures, there may be a cultural objection to organ donation and reception; however, there is no religious restriction on either donating or accepting organs. The patient should be asked for his/her preferences.

END OF LIFE

Death rituals vary considerably depending on culture.

In traditional Chinese culture, there are five funeral stages:

6. In the first stage, the dying person sees every member of his or her family before death. This is a *familial obligation*, and the patient should be provided with a private room to accommodate the potentially large number of visitors if possible.

7. The second stage is *announcement* of the death to the community.

8. The third stage is *bathing* the body with fresh water so that the deceased can pass into the next world comfortably; providers should ask ahead of time to determine whether or not the body should be washed in the hospital.

9. The fourth stage is called "*the Lamp to Light the Way*," in which family members place a plant-oil lamp at the feet of the corpse as mourners gather.

10. The fifth stage is *burial*. Traditionally, the deceased is not buried until resting in his/her house for three days.

Taoist or Confucian priests will likely be called to assist in these stages, depending on the religion of the deceased.

Confucius did not believe in life after death; he explained that because people cannot know what happens after death, they should concentrate their efforts on the living and rituals to be performed. His *Book of Rites* contains strict rules for rituals to be followed after death and explains in great detail how the body should be arranged, how mourners should behave, what mourners should wear, and more. The main purpose of Confucian rites is to secure peace for the soul of the deceased and to separate the living from the dead; this separation is necessary to protect the living and help the dead join their ancestors. Practitioners should discuss plans with the family to see which rites, if any, they wish to observe.

In contrast to Confucianism, Taoism teaches that the deceased can become supernatural if s/he cultivated a moral character during life. Taoist funerary rites have four main components, designed to help the deceased make his/her way in the afterlife:

- *Chanting scriptures.* The chanting of scriptures is arguably the most important funeral ritual; it is believed that this will release the dead from their suffering. The most common scriptures used during funerals are the *Book of Salvation,* the *Book of the Jade Emperor* and the *Book of the Three Officials.*

- *Water and land rituals.* The water and land rituals traditionally last seven days. During this time, an altar is built and elaborate rites are performed in order to pardon the guilt of the deceased; it is believed that this helps him/her to ascend into heaven or to have a good reincarnation.

- *Lighting and disposing of lanterns.* Traditionally, lanterns were lit at an altar, symbolizing the enlightenment of the deceased's soul; the lights were also believed to guide the deceased out of the realm of death. In honor of this tradition, Taoists may choose to light an oil lamp at the feet of the corpse. During the funeral, mourners may also place paper lamps in rivers or lakes. Taoist tradition teaches that people must pass through a dark river after death, and the water lanterns are believed to help the deceased pass over the river.

- *Feeding hungry ghosts.* Lastly, there are rituals for the feeding of hungry ghosts. Taoism teaches that there are some people who do not find everything they need to survive in the afterlife. If not fed, these hungry ghosts will feed off the energy and fear of the living. In order to placate them, a feeding ritual is performed that includes praying, chanting, and food offerings. The extent and extravagance of these ceremonies often depends on the wealth of the family.

Many Chinese and Chinese Americans mix elements from multiple religions into the funeral rites of the deceased. Thus, each family should be asked for their preference on how to handle the body.

FOR MORE READING: CHINESE FOLK RELIGION, CONFUCIANISM, AND TAOISM

Kraemer T. Cultural considerations for the Chinese culture. In: Latanzi JB, Purnell LD, eds. *Developing Cultural Competence in Physical Therapy Practice*. Philadelphia, PA: FA Davis. 2006:179-207.

Schott J, Henley A. Traditional Chinese culture. In: Schott J, Henley A, eds. *Culture, Religion and Childbearing in a Multiracial Society*. Oxford, UK: Butterworth-Heinemann. 1996: 257-267.

Shuang L. The funeral and Chinese culture. *J Pop Cult.* 1993; 27[2]: 113-120.

Tan A. Health and illness in the Asian population. In: Spector RE, ed. *Cultural Diversity in Health and Illness*. 6th ed. Upper Saddle River, NJ: Pearson Education. 2004: 209-229.

Tsai JN. Eye on religion: By the brush and by the sword: Daoist perspectives on the body, illness, and healing. *Southern Med J.* 2006; 99[12]: 1452-53.

9. American Indian & Alaska Native (AIAN) Religious Traditions

••••

Overview FAQ

1. When, where, and how did AIAN religious traditions originate?
Some scholars believe that the ancestors of AIANs migrated to North America from Asia more than 12,000 years ago, bringing with them a type of shamanism, a religion in which holy people mediate between the visible and spirit worlds. However, most AIAN tribal traditions hold that their ancestors were created in North America, and these beliefs have been passed on and adapted by subsequent generations.

Historically, AIAN religious and spiritual practices were completely integrated with day-to-day life and did not entail any special observances or times; no Indian language has a word that translates into "religion."

2. Do AIAN religious traditions have sacred texts? What are they called?
AIAN tribes pass on their beliefs through oral tradition rather than through written texts.

3. What are the core beliefs of AIAN religious traditions?
Though the beliefs and spiritual practices of AIANs vary by tribe and region, most believe that there is a Great Power or Spirit that underlies all creation.

Rather than emphasizing the primacy of human beings, most AIANs believe that all things in the universe are alive, contain a spirit within them, and should be valued accordingly. Special reverence and respect is given to the earth, which is believed to nourish and sustain life.

Often, certain individuals in the tribe are thought to have a special connection to the Great Power that enables them to mediate between the earthly world and the spirit world to provide healing and spiritual renewal for the good of the community. Most AIANs strive to live in balance and harmony with the material and spirit worlds; to do this is to "walk in the sacred way." How one carries this out is highly personal and often guided by dreams and visions. One's physical and spiritual health is dependent on proper actions and interactions with the spirit world.

4. What are the core practices of AIAN religious traditions?

AIAN rituals and practices vary greatly between tribes. In some tribes, prayer is spontaneous, while in others, prayers are memorized and recited verbatim. Despite these differences, for nearly all AIANs, prayer is more than just spoken word – it is a way of life that is necessary for maintaining a proper balance between the material and the spirit worlds.

Dance and drama are also commonly used to communicate with higher powers. These ceremonial dance-dramas can commemorate the past, symbolize the actions of powerful spirits, or dramatize the relationship between the natural and spiritual worlds. Performers often wear elaborate masks and costumes that represent the spirit world. Music also plays an important function during these rites and is believed to have supernatural power.

Another practice that is nearly universal among North Americans is the Sweat Lodge Ceremony, a purification ritual that precedes other important ceremonies. During a sweat ceremony, adherents sit in a small, heated chamber while a spiritual leader offers songs and prayers for healing and well-being. It is commonly believed that animal spirits are present throughout the ceremony.

5. What are the AIAN religious traditions' important holidays? How are they celebrated?

Although each tribe has different festivals that are celebrated throughout the year, most AIAN communities hold a world renewal ceremony annually in which the creation of the world is celebrated and rituals to promote order and harmony are performed. This celebration marks the beginning of the ritual year for many AIANs, and is followed by holidays throughout the year that honor different agricultural and natural cycles and celebrate humans' connection to the natural world.

These celebrations often include dance, song, prayer, music, sacrifice, and offering. They seek to restore balance on behalf of the entire world, not just for any particular tribe or for AIANs generally.

6. How many adherents of AIAN religious traditions are there in the United States? Are they located in a particular region?

Approximately 2.5 million people in the United States and Canada self-identify as AIAN. Of those, it is difficult to say how many practice a form of AIAN spirituality since it is a complex mix of both culture and religion. Those who live on or near ancestral lands are more likely to have preserved the religious practices of their ancestors. However, most AIANs, regardless of their location, follow at least some cultural and religious practices of their tribe.

7. What are the main sects or denominations within AIAN religious traditions?

There is no single "AIAN religion" since each tribe has its own set of beliefs and religious practices based on their particular history and culture. Non-AIANs may consider each tribe a denomination, but most AIANs would understand their spirituality as reflective of the belief system of their tribe rather than the sect of a larger religion. Additionally, many AIANs consider themselves ethnically and culturally AIAN while practicing other organized religions not indigenous to their tribes.

Some tribal communities have merged outside religious practices with tribal ceremonies. For example, the Pueblo community has integrated parts of Catholic observance into Pueblo ritual, and ceremonial dancers, drummers, and singers will attend Catholic mass and receive communion before beginning the Pueblo ceremony.

In addition to membership in their tribe, some AIANs are members of the Native American Church, a religious denomination developed in the early 20th century. Quannah Parker is credited with founding the religion after seeing a vision of Jesus Christ while consuming peyote, a southwestern cactus believed to have supernatural powers. Parker's teachings comprise the core beliefs of the Native American Church and include: peyote's personification as a God; Jesus as an AIAN cultural hero, a supreme God, and several lesser gods/spirits; and the Bible as a sacred text. The most important religious practice of those in the Church is the ritual consumption of peyote, which is viewed as a gift given to AIANs by the Creator.

· · · ·

Intersections with Health Care: FAQ

1. Do AIAN religious traditions have a particular view about what causes illness? Are there illness-related rituals?

Though there is great diversity of beliefs within AIAN religions, most teach that human health is dependent upon one's relation to the supernatural. Thus, illness can only be overcome when one regains proper balance with the forces of the universe. To achieve this balance, AIANs often turn to the medical practitioners in their own communities before seeking Western medical help.

Depending on the tribe, illness may be attributed to such varied causes as displeasing the cosmos, disturbing plant or animal life, or neglecting the celestial bodies. Once the cause is determined, special divination ceremonies may be performed. These ceremonies vary from tribe to tribe, but can include meditation, trances, sacred singing, and purification rituals. Herbal treatments are also often prescribed.

2. Do AIAN religious traditions prescribe a particular type of dress?

Many AIANs believe that certain objects are sacred, including stones, feathers, antlers, fur, claws, shells, and crystals. These sacred objects are usually placed inside cloth or leather pouches, called medicine bags, which may be worn on the body. If a patient is wearing such an item, it should not be touched or removed without consent. If removal is necessary, the item should either be given to the patient to hold, placed near the patient, or given to a family member.

3. Are there any prayer or ritual observances that are likely to occur during the patient's stay?

Some AIANs may wish to hold healing ceremonies while a patient is in the hospital. If possible, privacy is appreciated. Though there are countless traditions among tribes, some are more prevalent than others. These include: smudging the patient with sage, cedar, and sweet grass for purification; ceremonially painting the patient's face in preparation for surgery or death; pipe ceremonies; visiting community members who chant, sing, drum, or rattle; purification ceremonies that involve praying and calling ancestors for help; and placing crystals or sacred stones on the patient's body.

4. Do AIAN religious traditions have hygiene or washing requirements?

It is important that health care practitioners check with the patient or his/her family before cutting or shaving hair, since some tribes associate this with mourning.

5. Are there any dietary restrictions?

Some AIAN tribes encourage the consumption of traditional food during the period leading up to important ceremonies; the practice and the foods associated with it vary by tribe.

Fasting is a common spiritual practice for some AIANs. It is often done to prepare for ceremonies. If a patient is unable to fast for health reasons, close family or friends may fast on his/her behalf.

6. Are there any medications, treatments, or procedures that AIAN religious tradition adherents cannot accept?

Many AIAN traditions teach that pain is something to be endured. Thus, health care providers may face resistance when attempting to prescribe pain medication. Additional resistance may spring from the patient's desire to treat the illness with traditional herbal medicines. Some AIANs are skeptical of Western medical treatment and may be reluctant to share what herbal remedies they are using.

Patients may be especially reticent to take medication at the end of life, as some believe that it is important to die with a clear and open mind.

7. Can patients from AIAN religious traditions see providers of the opposite sex?

Some AIANs may prefer providers of the same sex; however, this is typically more of a personal preference that varies from patient to patient.

8. Can adherents of AIAN religious traditions donate organs or accept donor organs?

Some AIAN tribes believe that the whole body must be present in order to enter into the next world. Those holding this belief may be unreceptive to organ donation.

9. Should I consult anyone other than the patient when seeking informed consent or other patient decisions?

Extended family is very important for many AIANs, so an individual's illness often concerns the entire family. Decision making structures among AIAN traditions vary according to both the individual and the kinship organization of his/her tribe. In most tribes, the elders of the community are highly revered and should be consulted. Frequently, this individual will be an older woman.

Due to the historical misuse of signed documents to dispossess the AIAN population, some may be resistant to signing informed consent agreements or advanced directives.

10. What are AIAN religious traditions' views on reproductive health and family planning? Are contraceptives okay? What about abortion? Voluntary sterilization?

Traditionally, AIAN women used medicines and herbs to take care of their reproductive health, including contraception and abortion; this was accepted by both AIAN men and women. However, these beliefs have not historically been respected by the federal agency charged with AIAN health care.

The Indian Health Service (IHS) is the federal agency that is responsible for providing health care to all AIANs. In 2005, the IHS served approximately 50% of AIANs. Since it is a federal agency, abortions are extremely rare, despite the high rate of sexual assault in this population (the U.S. Department of Justice estimates that one in three AIAN women will be raped or sexually assaulted during her lifetime—a rate $3\frac{1}{2}$ times greater than among all other racial groups).

Sterilization is also a very sensitive topic for many AIANs. The U.S. government admitted in the mid-1970s that the IHS had performed several thousand sterilizations on women without proper consent. Most AIAN rights activists consider the involuntary sterilization an act of population control on their community.

Thus, the reproductive health of AIAN women should be handled with extreme sensitivity to both the traditional beliefs of the population and to their historical mistreatment.

11. Are there particular beliefs or rituals concerning pregnancy and birth? What about postpartum women? What about women who have miscarried?

Some AIAN women prefer to use a female relative as a birth attendant and may want to use special herbs and teas during labor. It is also common for special songs to be sung and incense burned in honor of a birth. The newborn may be smudged with special plants or herbs.

The family should be asked if it would like the placenta and umbilical cord saved. Some will save the umbilical cord throughout their lifetimes, reminding them of their connections both to their mothers and to Mother Earth.

12. Are there end-of-life rituals or beliefs I need to know about?

Discussing terminal prognoses or Do Not Resuscitate orders may be difficult with some AIANs, since negative thoughts and words about one's health are believed to hasten death. When discussing fatal diseases or illnesses, the health care provider may wish to speak in the third person. Speaking of it directly may inadvertently indicate that the health care provider does not value the patient's life.

Visitation customs for AIAN patients vary from tribe to tribe. Some wish to avoid contact with the dying, while others believe that it is important to be at a person's side throughout the last hours of his/her life. Whether family members are present or not, mourning is often done in private and away from the patient.

Many AIANs believe that they rejoin their ancestors at death, and patients who are nearing death may report visits and conversations with deceased family members.

It is common for the extended family and community members to bring food to the patient, as it is seen as a necessary aid as one prepares for the spirit's journey.

13. What should be done with the body after death?

Because each tribe has its own traditions, providers should not make assumptions. As a general rule, the body should not be moved until the family has been consulted about its particular tradition.

Otherwise, customs vary by tribe. Some may want a window left open to allow the soul to exit the room. Others may want the patient's body oriented to a cardinal direction, for ceremonial objects to be placed on the body, or to dress the body in special clothing. Many tribes cut a piece of hair from the deceased. For some AIANs, it is important that the name of the deceased not be spoken, as this may hold the person's spirit in limbo and delay his/her journey into the next world; for others, the name of the deceased is spoken repeatedly as part of a ceremonial ritual.

• • • •

AIAN Traditions: Intersections with Health Care

The blanket term "American Indian/Alaska Natives" (AIANs) covers a vast array of people, some of whom refer to themselves as "Indians": there are 2.4 million AIANs in the United States, and over 550 federally recognized tribes, each with their own unique understanding of how humans relate to the earth and the cosmos as well as their own beliefs and practices around illness. A comprehensive overview of the beliefs and practices of every AIAN tribe is not possible; thus, this manual endeavors to:

1. Provide an overview of the beliefs and practices that *are* shared across tribes;

2. Provide an overview of the beliefs and practices of the Native American Church, which is a syncretic blend of AIAN and Christian beliefs; and

3. Identify the areas in which providers will need to seek additional information from their patients.

It is important to note that many tribes refer to themselves with their indigenous names rather than the names they were assigned during the Colonial period; for example, "Navajo" is a Spanish word, and the tribe itself uses the indigenous name, "Diné."

CAUSES OF ILLNESS & HEALING RITUALS

Though there is a great diversity of beliefs within AIAN religions, most teach that humans' health depends on their relationship with the supernatural. In the AIAN worldview, a person is a small piece of a larger, interconnected world, and both bodily and mental health are inextricably connected to one's harmony with the cosmos. Thus, illness is only overcome when one regains proper balance with the forces of the universe. To achieve this balance, AIANs may turn to the medical practitioners in their own communities before seeking Western medical help.

The causes of illness may be attributed to such varied origins as displeasing the cosmos, abandoning tribal traditions, disturbing plant or animal life, or neglecting the celestial bodies. In almost all cases, the causes of illness are believed to be supernatural. Traditional healers possess the supernatural powers necessary to address them. These healers are called medicine men and women, shamans, or singers, and have different sacred gifts, including:

- The ability to *see* what caused the illness;
- The power to *rid* the patient of the evil causing the illness;
- The ability to *care* for the soul and to send guardian spirits to restore a lost soul; and
- The ability to *heal* through the use of song and/or herbal medicines.

Once the cause has been determined, special divination ceremonies may be performed. These ceremonies vary from tribe to tribe, but can include meditation, trances, sacred singing, and purification rituals. Once the proper rituals have been performed, a traditional healer often prescribes herbal treatments.

Many AIANs believe that stating aloud that a person has an illness or particular prognosis will cause it to occur. In speaking about illness and health conditions, therefore, it may be useful to speak in the third person.

DRESS & MODESTY

Unlike some religious traditions, most AIAN tribes do not prescribe particular types of dress for men and women. The best way to learn whether a particular patient has any dress or modesty-related requirements is to ask him/her.

Although a patient may not have a particular type of required dress, some AIANs do wear sacred objects. Items considered sacred include stones, feathers, antlers, fur, claws, and cloth or leather pouches, which may be worn or placed in a special part of the hospital room.

The pouches are called medicine bags or bundles and contain sacred objects such as shells, stones, crystal, feathers, and/or tobacco. Medicine bags may belong to the individual patient, or belong to his/her family or tribe. If the patient is wearing such an item, it should not be touched or removed without the patient's consent, because its possession is believed to be both a great honor and a serious responsibility. If removal is necessary, the item should be treated with the utmost respect and either given to the patient to hold, placed near the patient, or given to a trusted family member.

Tribes who engage in dance rituals are likely to wear elaborate masks and costumes representing the spirit world. These items have great spiritual significance and are not likely to be seen outside of rituals performed within the privacy of the communities. However, if any patient has a mask or costume in his/her room, it should not be touched without the patient's consent and should be handled carefully if consent is given.

GENDER & MODESTY

Some AIANs may prefer to be treated by providers of the same sex. This preference will likely vary from patient to patient. Providers should ask each individual patient about his/her preferences.

PRAYERS & RITUAL OBSERVANCES

Some AIANs may wish to hold healing ceremonies while the patient is in the hospital. In many tribes, these healing rituals are observed only by those within the tribe, so that strict privacy is appreciated if at all possible. Because the most sacred traditions are often passed orally from traditional healer to traditional healer, information on healing practices can be limited.

Though there are a variety of ceremonies performed according to the tradition of each AIAN tribe, some are more prevalent than others. Some of the most common ceremonies include:

- Smudging the patient with sacred plants like sage, cedar, and sweet grass for purification and to bring about an openness to healing;

- Ceremonially painting the patient's face in preparation for surgery or death;

- A pipe ceremony, which a patient may wish to conduct in the hospital;

- Visiting community members who chant, sing, drum, or rattle. These sounds are believed to aid in the process of recovery, and remind the patient that s/he is not alone;

- Medicine lodge, a purification ceremony involving prayers and calling of ancestors for help. This may be requested before surgery; and

- Placement of crystals or sacred stones on a person's body.

All of these rituals are aimed at helping to put the patient in the right state of mind for healing. Some may conflict with health care facility policies. For example, a pipe ceremony might not be possible in a non-smoking facility. While it may not be feasible to perform some ceremonies in a hospital setting, patients will appreciate efforts to accommodate their religious needs.

In addition to these traditional rituals, members of the AIAN Church commonly perform the peyote ritual. The AIAN Church, founded in the 1890s, blends Christianity and tribal belief systems. Peyote, a fruit from a southwestern cactus, acts as a mild hallucinogen when ingested. The plant migrated from Central to North America in the 15th century and is used as an aid to healing, as a way to cleanse evil spirits, and to commune with the spirit world. Members of the AIAN Church compare their use of peyote to the use of sacramental wine in Christian communion.

In peyote rituals, church members ingest the plant and have all-night worship meetings while under the influence of the hallucinogen. The ritual commonly begins at 8:00 p.m. on a Saturday and includes prayer, peyote songs, and individual contemplation. It ends with breakfast on Sunday morning.

Consumption of peyote is legal under U.S. law, but only when done under the auspices of the AIAN Church. Despite its legality within the Church, health care providers should be aware that it is only legal if it is part of a religious ritual, and local law enforcement agencies may be reluctant to recognize its legality. Communication between patients and the health care provider is crucial if patients wish to be part of a peyote ritual while in the hospital. Often, it is suggested that AIAN Church members practice the ritual outside of the confines of a hospital, whenever possible, to reduce the possible legal objections.

HYGIENE AND WASHING REQUIREMENTS

There are no general rules around hygiene or washing for AIAN tribes.

It *is* important that health care practitioners check with the patient or his/her family members before cutting or shaving hair, because some tribes associate uncut hair with mourning. If a person is in mourning and does not want his/her hair cut despite medical necessity, the reasons should be explained to the patient and the least amount necessary cut.

DIETARY REQUIREMENTS

As a general rule, most AIAN tribes don't have the type of food restrictions found in many other religions—for example, Judaism's kashruth requirements or Islam and halal—although there are a few exceptions to this generality. What AIAN tribes often have are food-related beliefs and practices that often come into play in the health care environment.

Some AIAN tribes encourage the consumption of traditional food during the period leading up to important ceremonies or events. Family and friends may wish to bring the patient meals; this should be allowed unless there is a medical contraindication.

Fasting is also a common spiritual practice for some AIANs. It is often done as a traditional part of the preparation for certain ceremonies. If the patient is unable to fast for health reasons, close family or friends sometimes fast on his/her behalf. Different patients may interpret the fasting requirements differently. Providers should discuss fasting with the patient and his/her family to ensure that the patient will not cause himself/herself additional harm by fasting during illness or recovery and that fasting will not interfere substantially with compliance with needed medical treatment (i.e. because the patient may not want to orally ingest pills, capsules, or liquid medications).

In addition, some tribes believe that certain categories of food should be eaten during certain life stages. Pregnancy, in particular, has a variety of food prescriptions and taboos. Many tribes recommend that an expectant mother eat "strong" foods to ensure a healthy pregnancy; which foods are considered strong may vary, although this often includes corn. Fatty, salty, or sweet foods may also be prohibited during certain illnesses or rituals; providers should ask the patient and his/her family whether they are observing any particular rituals requiring food restrictions or imbibing during times of illness.

MEDICATION, TREATMENT, AND PROCEDURE RESTRICTIONS

Many AIAN traditions teach that pain is something to be endured. Thus, the health care provider may face resistance when attempting to give a patient medication.

Additional resistance may spring from a AIAN patient's desire to treat illness with traditional herbal medicines. Some AIANs are skeptical of Western medical treatment and may be reluctant to share which herbal medications they are taking with Western health care providers. Providers should make clear to the patient that traditional remedies are welcome, but that it is important that they are disclosed to ensure that there are no negative reactions between the traditional and the Western treatments. In addition, patients may be especially resistant to taking medication at the end of their lives, as some believe that it is important to die with a clear and open mind.

Historically, there is a high rate of alcohol and substance abuse among AIANs and sensitivity to the stereotypes that accompany this phenomenon often make it a difficult subject to discuss. The issue of substance abuse should be approached carefully, when it is suspected. Additionally, some AIANs may be reluctant to take any medication, out of fear that it will be addictive. In these cases, good communication about the benefits and risks will be helpful between the health care provider and patients.

Some AIAN patients will not want their photographs taken without permission. If X-rays, CT scans, MRIs, or any other type of imagery is necessary for patient care, the health care provider should take time to explain to the patient the purpose of the procedure and the type of images that will be taken.

AIAN patients should be asked if their tribe has any beliefs surrounding amputated body parts. For some tribes, there is a religious requirement to return an amputated part to the patient so that it may be blessed and buried or cremated with the patient; this can be important because some tribes teach that the body must be buried intact.

ORGAN DONATION

Some AIAN tribes believe that the whole body must be present in order to enter into the next world. Those holding this belief may be unreceptive to organ donation. Moreover, if amputation is necessary, the patient may request that the body part be blessed and either cremated or buried soon after removal.

INFORMED CONSENT & PATIENT DECISION MAKING

The extended family is very important for many AIANs, so an individual's illness may concern the entire family. Decision making guidelines among tribes vary according to both the individual and the kinship structure of his/her tribe. In most tribes, the elders of the community are highly revered and should be consulted for major health care decisions. Frequently, this individual will be an older woman in the community.

Due to the historical misuse of signed documents to dispossess the AIAN population, some may be resistant to signing informed consent agreements or advanced directives at all.

REPRODUCTIVE HEALTH & FAMILY PLANNING

Traditionally, AIAN women used medicines and herbs to take care of their reproductive health, including contraception and abortion (within most native languages, there is no translation for "abortion"). Women were understood to be the keepers of their own bodies, and it was usually women who maintained the knowledge of herbs and techniques used in reproductive health and birth. This state of things was accepted by both AIAN men and women. However, these beliefs have not historically been respected by the federal agency charged with AIAN health care.

The Indian Health Service (IHS) is the federal agency that is responsible for providing health care to all AIANs. In 2005, the IHS served approximately 50% of AIANs. Because it is a federal agency, abortions are extremely rare, despite a high rate of sexual assault in this population (the U.S. Department of Justice estimates that one in three AIAN women will be raped or sexually assaulted during her lifetime—a rate 3½ times greater than among all other racial groups).

Sterilization is also a very sensitive topic for many AIANs. The U.S. government admitted in the mid-1970s that the IHS had performed several thousand sterilizations, both surgical and with hormonal implants, on women without proper consent. Many AIAN rights activists consider this involuntary sterilization a violation and an act of enforced population control targeted to their community.

Thus, issues involving the reproductive health of AIAN women should be handled with extreme sensitivity to both the traditional beliefs of the population and to their historical mistreatment.

PREGNANCY & BIRTH

Some AIAN women may prefer to have a female relative as their birth attendant; they may also want to use special herbs and teas during labor. Providers should ask whether a laboring woman has used an herbal remedy or tea.

It is common for special songs to be performed at the time of birth, and incense may be burned in honor of the birth. The newborn may be smudged with special plants or herbs. Again, providers may need to ask about these herbs and make a determination as to whether or not they are safe for a newborn. If there is an issue, this should be clearly explained to the mother and the family and alternative herbs or rituals explored.

The family should be asked if they would like the placenta and umbilical cord saved. Some AIANs will retain the umbilical cords of their children throughout their lifetimes as a reminder of their connection to their mothers and to Mother Earth. Postpartum, the mother and infant may rest inside for twenty days or until the umbilical cord falls off.

Many AIAN traditions have naming ceremonies in which the baby is formally initiated into the tribe and the larger community. It is believed that names have the power to shape an individual's future and they are chosen carefully, often by an elder of the family or tribe. Among some tribes, it is believed that the souls of ancestors are reborn into the tribe and children may be named accordingly. In other tribes, names signify social rank or have a meaning into which elders hope the child will grow.

Often, girls receive a birth name that they will keep throughout their lives. Boys sometimes get new names as they enter into different stages of their lives. Medical records should reflect all the names given to a child.

END OF LIFE

Discussing terminal prognoses or Do Not Resuscitate orders may be difficult with some AIANs because expressing aloud negative thoughts and words about one's health is believed to hasten death. When discussing fatal diseases or illnesses, the health care provider may wish to speak of the issue in the third person—speaking of it directly may inadvertently indicate to the patient that the health care provider does not value his/her life.

Despite these beliefs, there is a general acceptance of death as a natural and inevitable part of the cycle of life. Many will expect their bodies to return to Mother Earth and for their souls to move on in the next world, where they will join ancestors. Accordingly, patients who are nearing death may report visits and conversations with deceased family members.

AIAN customs around visiting the ill vary from tribe to tribe. Some may wish to avoid contact with the dying, while others believe that it is important to be at the patient's side throughout the last hours of his/her life. Whether family members are present or not, mourning is often done in private and away from the patient. It is common for the extended family and members of the community to bring food to a patient, as it is seen as a necessary aid as one prepares for the spirit's journey.

Additionally, many AIANs believe that death should be met with a clear and open mind. Therefore, they may be reluctant to take any medications. This should be discussed carefully with the patient. Often, it is helpful to bring other members of the tribe into this conversation, because it is common for health care decisions to be made communally.

Post death customs vary by tribe. Some may want a window left open to allow the soul to leave at death. Others may want the patient's body to be oriented to a cardinal direction, or for ceremonial objects to be placed on the body, or they may wish to dress the body in special clothing. Many tribes cut a piece of hair from the deceased. For some AIANs, it is important that the name of the deceased not be spoken, as this may hold the person's spirit in limbo and delay his/her journey into the next world; for others, the name of the deceased is spoken repeatedly as part of a ceremonial ritual. Each tribe has its own tradition and assumptions should not be made. As a general rule, however, the body should not be moved until the family has been consulted about their particular tradition.

Diné/Navajo end-of-life beliefs require some special consideration. Traditionally, speaking of death is unacceptable, as this is believed to hasten death. In addition, Diné tradition teaches that the good parts of the person's soul become part of the harmony and balance of the universe after death, while the bad parts remain on earth. The evil parts left behind have the power to harm the living. The Diné destroy the clothes and possessions of the deceased and are careful to never speak the person's name, as uttering a name might attract a wandering ghost and threaten the health of those left behind.

Health care providers working with Navajo patients and their families should avoid speaking directly about death before the patient passes. After the patient dies, the provider should not mention his/her name.

FOR MORE READING: AIAN RELIGIOUS TRADITIONS

Cochran TM, Cross PS. Cultural considerations for American Indian cultures. In: Lattanzi JB, Purnell LD, eds. *Developing Cultural Competence in Physical Therapy Practice*. Philadelphia, PA: FA Davis. 2006: 238-259.

Hartz PR. *Native American Religions*. New York, NY: Facts on File. 2004.

Hultkrantz A. Health, religion, and medicine in native North American traditions. In: Sullivan LE, ed. *Healing and Restoring: Health and Medicine in the World's Religious Traditions*. New York, NY: MacMillan. 1989: 327-358.

Murphy JM. *Working the Spirit: Ceremonies of the African Diaspora*. Boston, MA: Beacon Press. 1994.

Spector RE. Health and illness in the American Indian and Alaska native population. In: *Cultural Diversity in Health & Illness*. Upper Saddle River, NJ: Pearson Education. 2004: 185-207.

Taylor EJ. AIAN religiosity. In: *Spiritual Care: Nursing Theory, Research, and Practice*. Upper Saddle River, NJ: Prentice Hall. 2002: 239-240.

Tom-Orme L. Transcultural nursing and health care among AIAN peoples. In: Leininger M, McFarland MR, eds. *Transcultural Nursing: Concepts, Theories, Research and Practice*. 3rd ed. New York, NY: McGraw-Hill. 2002: 429-441.

PART 3: RELIGIONS OF THE WORLD & THEIR APPLICATIONS TO HEALTH CARE

10. Afro-Caribbean Religious Traditions
. . . .

Overview FAQ

1. When, where, and how did the Afro-Caribbean religions originate?
From the 15th through 19th centuries, the Caribbean basin was the site of an extended encounter between the Old and New Worlds, as Spain, Holland, Portugal, France, and the British Isles competed against each other for control of the Caribbean islands, as well as Central and South America. The major European colonies in the region include Jamaica, Haiti, Cuba, Trinidad, Puerto Rico, Martinique, Curacao, Grenada, St. Lucia, and many smaller islands, as well as countries such as Belize, Honduras, Brazil, Suriname, French Guiana, and Guyana. In addition to enslaving the native population, the colonizers brought Africans from Central and Western Africa as slaves to the New World and sought to convert them to Christianity.

In each colony, Christian religions (such as the Anglican and Dutch Reformed churches and the national Catholic churches of France, Portugal, and Spain) became the state religions. Christian sects other than these state churches suffered persecution and non-Christian religions such as Islam, AIAN religions, and traditional African religions were often actively suppressed. Nonetheless, some indigenous Caribbean and African populations resisted conversion and held onto their own religious beliefs, while incorporating elements of Christianity. This process resulted in the creation of a variety of religious forms that incorporate elements from indigenous Caribbean beliefs and West and Central African religions, as well as institutional and popular forms of Christianity and even folk religious traditions practiced in Europe.

These religious traditions are syncretic. That is, they are traditions that have beliefs and practices from different religions and/or cultures and interact with one another to form a new belief system that incorporates and reconciles aspects of both.

Major Afro-Caribbean traditions include Candomblé, Palo Mayombe, Santería, Vodoun, Rastafarianism, and Revivalism.

2. Do Afro-Caribbean religions have sacred texts? What are they called?
In the Afro-Caribbean religious groups with the strongest Christian influence, such as Revivalism and Rastafarianism, the Bible is a central sacred text. Rastafarians in

particular view the Bible as a sacred text that Christians in general and the colonizing European churches in particular have willfully misinterpreted and misunderstood in order to oppress and exploit people of African descent.

In these traditions, the Bible also plays additional roles that are unknown to most North American Christians. For example, some Revivalist churches view the Bible not only as a source of doctrine, salvation, and divine revelation, but also as a book of magic, with the Books of Psalms and Revelations being especially potent sources of magical power for the person who knows how to use them correctly.

Some traditions also venerate the writings of key leaders. Rastafarianism utilizes the writings of Marcus Garvey as sacred texts, while Caribbean Spiritists sometimes use the works of Spiritism's French founder, Allan Kardec (aka Hyppolite Rivail), as sacred texts, including his *Selected Prayers*, *Book of the Medium*, and *Book of Spirits*.

Santería, Candomblé, Palo Mayombe, and Vodoun, although influenced by Catholicism and incorporating some Christian concepts and symbols, do not utilize the Bible as a sacred text. The most important sacred literature in these traditions are orally transmitted songs, stories, and prayers.

3. What are the core beliefs of Afro-Caribbean religions?

Although there are specific beliefs unique to each Afro-Caribbean religious tradition, they all share a common worldview.

God, an array of other spirits, human beings, and the natural world constitute a single interdependent reality. The names of God and the major deities and spirits vary among traditions:

Religion	Supreme being	Major Deities or Spirits	Spirits of the Dead
Candomblé	Olodumare	Orixas, Vodouns, Nkisis	Eguns
Santería	Olodumare, Olorun	Orishas	Eguns, Los Muertos
Vodoun	Bon Dye	Lwas	Lwas
Palo Mayombe	Nzambi	Mpungu	Nkisi, Mfumbe

Afro-Caribbean religions teach that the Supreme Being and spirits are interdependent and do not live in a world apart from humanity. Rather, the material and spiritual worlds are inseparable and interpenetrate one another. Humans and other natural objects are believed to be both natural and divine—participating in and influencing the spiritual world. As a result, a major focus of concern for believers is how to access various kinds of spiritual power.

These religions basically accept the world as it is, though they believe that the world can be made better and that the situations of individual people and groups can be improved. Although they all believe in reincarnation, the emphasis is not on future lives, but rather on personal and communal fulfillment in the present life. For their adherents, then, religion is the resource for dealing successfully with the physical, social, psychological, familial, spiritual, and financial obstacles they experience in life. These problems may be overcome through rituals that make use of the powers that are available in the natural world and in the various spirits they worship.

4. What are the core practices of Afro-Caribbean religions?

Although the particulars of practice vary among traditions, the main ways in which believers practice fall into a few broad categories.

- **Altars and devotions**: The daily routines of members include devotions practiced at altars in their homes. Adherents pray before an altar dedicated to one or more of the deities they worship and leave offerings of flowers, incense, water, or alcoholic beverages, and occasionally small sacrificial animals consecrated by a priest.

- **Divination**: Divination, where deities speak through human priests, is a core practice in Santería, Candomblé, and in some varieties of Palo Mayombe. Devotees approach priests with a problem, and divination allows the priest to diagnose its causes. Although Vodoun does not make use of divination techniques of this sort, initiation into the highest ranks of the Vodoun priesthood is believed to grant the power of clairvoyance.

- **Ceremonial Spirit Possession**: While Santería, Candomblé, Palo Mayombe, and Vodoun are not congregational religions, there are occasional semi-public ceremonies that bring large numbers of worshippers together. These are typically religious services in which the main activities are singing religious songs accompanied by drumming and dancing. The practices of singing, dancing, and drumming together call upon the religion's deities and invite them to visit the ceremony by taking over the body of one or more of the priests. Once possession occurs, the deity is dressed in special clothes and interacts with worshippers before departing. Ceremonies usually end with a closing ritual followed by a communal meal, which is shared with the deities by placing food in front of their altars.

- **Healing**: Healing constitutes a major focus of these religions. Whether a problem is social, psychological, or physical, devotees make use of herbal medicine, ritual healing, folk psychiatry, and counseling provided by their spiritual leaders. Some problems may also be believed to be the result of sorcery, and a portion of any healer's work is dedicated to combating the effects of such sorcery.

5. What are Afro-Caribbean religions' important holidays? How are they celebrated?

Because the religions of Candomblé, Santería, Palo Mayombe, and Vodoun developed in societies in which Catholicism was the state religion, the religions have evolved a system of correspondences that links their own deities with specific Catholic saints. These holidays differ somewhat by country, because some saints are the patron saints of particular countries and their holidays have both religious significance and nationalist components to them. For example, the celebration of Our Lady of Cobre, the patron saint of Cuba, corresponds with the celebration and recognition of the Santerían deity Oshún.

In other cases, American holidays have been treated in the same way. This is the case with Halloween. Among Vodoun worshippers in the United States, Halloween is now an occasion for ceremonies directed at Baron Samedi and the Guedes and Lwas, who are associated with the dead and graveyards.

The more public celebrations on saints' days follow the pattern of drum/dance/possession feats described earlier; private observances related to an individual's relationship to a particular deity are celebrated at home with sacrifices, offerings, and divination.

6. How many adherents of Afro-Caribbean religions are there in the United States? Are they located in a particular region?

According to the 2000 US Census, there are approximately 1.6 million Afro-Caribbeans living in the United States. Of these, it is extremely difficult to determine how many actively practice Afro-Caribbean syncretic religions. The Afro-Caribbean population is most prominent in Miami, New York City, Chicago, New Orleans, Los Angeles, and Boston.

7. What are the main sects or denominations within Afro-Caribbean religions?

Though Santería, Candomblé, Vodoun, and Palo Mayombe are diverse and members can and do differentiate between varying forms of practice among them, there are no prominent, formalized divisions.

• • • •

Intersections with Health Care: FAQ

1. Do Afro-Caribbean religious traditions have a particular view about what causes illness? Are there illness-related rituals?

In Afro-Caribbean religions, illness is traditionally attributed to an imbalance in relationships with the living, the dead and/or spirits. Healing rituals (which are kept largely secret from non-adherents) focus on restoring balance; many spiritual leaders are regarded as healers and will recommend certain rituals in addition to prescribing remedies made from herbs, spices, and roots. Despite belief in the efficacy of natural remedies, however, the relationship between traditional healing and Western medicine is generally viewed as complementary.

2. Do Afro-Caribbean religious traditions prescribe a particular type of dress for men or women?

Generally, there is no religious dress that is worn on a daily basis, although extravagant outfits may accompany rituals. Some Afro-Caribbean patients may choose to wear charms or amulets that are believed to ward off evil spirits; these should not be removed without consent.

3. Are there any prayer or ritual observances that are likely to occur during the patient's stay?

Afro-Caribbean religious practitioners are often protective of their rituals, making it difficult to give specific examples of what a health care provider might encounter and highlighting the need to offer privacy for prayer and ritual observances whenever possible. Patients may bring in special food, icons, candles, or natural objects (e.g., rocks, sticks, etc), none of which should be touched without patient consent.

4. Do Afro-Caribbean religious traditions have hygiene or washing requirements?

Hygiene and personal cleanliness are very important to most people from Afro-Caribbean traditions. It is important to provide patients with washing facilities, particularly postnatal women. Some Afro-Caribbean patients may wish to add an antiseptic or other substance recommended by a religious leader to their bath water.

5. Are there any dietary restrictions?

Typically, there are no explicit, universal dietary restrictions. However, some may ascribe healing properties to food and wish to maintain a diet that they believe provides spiritual balance; others may want to eat foods associated with the particular spirits that they have sworn to serve. Many patients will prefer to eat food brought by friends and relatives.

6. Are there any medications, treatments, or procedures that adherents of Afro-Caribbean religious traditions cannot accept?

Generally, there will be no objections to particular medications, treatments, or procedures. However, patients may wish to combine medication prescribed by a Western medical practitioner with herbal remedies prescribed by a traditional healer.

7. Can patients from Afro-Caribbean religious traditions see providers of the opposite sex?

Many patients prefer to be seen by a provider of the same sex, although for cultural rather than religious reasons.

8. Can adherents of Afro-Caribbean religious traditions donate organs or accept donor organs?

Organ donation and reception are generally permissible, although each patient should be consulted.

9. Should I consult anyone other than the patient when seeking informed consent?

Close bonds between immediate and extended family members are common in Afro-Caribbean culture. Patients will often want older and respected members of the family to be involved in decision making. Some may even expect bad news (e.g., poor prognoses) to be shared first with the oldest immediate family member. Providers may wish to clarify that prognoses are given to the patient first unless s/he explicitly requests otherwise.

10. What are Afro-Caribbean religious traditions' views on reproductive health and family planning? Are contraceptives okay? What about abortion? Voluntary sterilization?

For most Afro-Caribbean women, there is a strong social pressure to give birth. In most cases, the husband prefers to be included in discussions of contraception or sterilization. However, it is not unusual for women to make the decisions on contraception and family planning. Culturally, abortion is largely discouraged and is accompanied by a social stigma.

In Haitian Vodoun, there is a specific belief surrounding pregnant women called *perdition* (*pedisyon*). It is believed that during pregnancy, the blood that normally exits during a woman's period is held in the womb as nourishment for the child. In perdition, the nourishing blood bypasses the fetus, arresting the pregnancy. A fetus may stay in a state of arrested growth for years until it can "untie" itself from perdition. Providers discussing issues around menstruation or infertility with adherents of Haitian Vodoun should be aware that this may be an issue for patients; it may also mean that patients with menstrual irregularities may delay seeking treatment.

11. Are there particular beliefs or rituals concerning pregnancy and birth? What about postpartum women? What about women who have miscarried?

Women may take herbs believed to enhance the health of the fetus during their pregnancies. Pregnant and postnatal women are thought to be especially vulnerable to supernaturally influenced health problems and many choose to avoid strenuous activities.

In some Afro-Caribbean cultures, women believe that they must avoid any activities that might cause a chill. For a few days after birth, a mother might be reticent to bathe or wash her hair.

Amulets or charms may be placed around a baby's wrist to ward off evil spirits.

12. Are there end-of-life rituals or beliefs I need to know about?

Given the importance of extended family and faith communities, an Afro-Caribbean patient is likely to receive a large number of visitors if death appears to be imminent. Many will not be restrained in their expression of mourning. A space for visitors to congregate and privacy during visitation would be appreciated.

13. What should be done with the body after death?

There are elaborate rituals in Afro-Caribbean religions surrounding death, many of which are not shared openly with the public. For this reason, it is important to work closely with family members to determine the most appropriate actions to be taken after death.

PART 3: RELIGIONS OF THE WORLD & THEIR APPLICATIONS TO HEALTH CARE

• • • •

Afro-Caribbean Religious Traditions: Intersections with Health Care

Afro-Caribbean religious traditions have no central religious authorities and no religious literature that is widely available. Because of their histories of persecution during the Colonial period and afterward, and because contemporary society and media continue to demonize them, there is a high level of secrecy around their beliefs and practices. Traditionally only priests, other initiates, and active devotees in a tradition take part in rituals and worship. Given the privacy surrounding these beliefs and rituals, little is publicly known about them and it is difficult to provide a comprehensive guide to what a health care provider might encounter. This section aims to:

1. Provide clear answers where they can be provided; and

2. Help providers understand areas in which further exploration with a particular patient might be necessary.

Quick answers for many questions that arise when caring for an Afro-Caribbean patient may be found in the FAQ. For more in-depth explanations, consult the appropriate section below.

CAUSES OF ILLNESS & HEALING RITUALS

Religious rituals and healing practices cannot be neatly separated in most Afro-Caribbean religions. There is no strong distinction made between spiritual well-being and physical health, or between physical illness and personal or social misfortune. All may be attributed to spiritual forces, even if these spiritual causes are mediated by natural or social influences. For example, if one individual loses a job and another contracts an illness, it is highly likely that both individuals will believe that their situation stems from spiritual aspects of their own lives as well as their relationships to deities, ancestors, and living people who may have used spiritual forces against them.

The cause of illness is traditionally attributed to an imbalance in one's relationships with the living, the dead, and/or spirits. Depending on the tradition, spirits have different names:

- In *Palo Mayombe*, they are called *Mpungu*.

- In *Santería*, they are called *Orishas* and *eguns*.

- In *Vodoun*, they are called *Lwas*.

- In *Candomblé*, they may be called *Orixás*, *Vodouns*, *Nkisis*, or *eguns*.

Healing rituals involve channeling the power of the spirits. This may be done through divination, offerings, chanting, prayer, manufacturing medicines, or other rituals.

Most Afro-Caribbean spiritual leaders are also healers with extensive knowledge of medicinal plants and traditional healing practices and rituals. Once a healer determines the nature and cause of an illness, s/he will recommend the appropriate rituals and other treatments; these may include remedies made from herbs, spices, oils, foods, animal parts, and other substances, as well as prayers, offerings, sacrifices, baths, or other ritual procedures.

When the spiritual leader of Afro-Caribbean traditions is an elder member of the family, they may be among the first people consulted when an illness is recognized. In addition, a network comprised of the devotees attached to a particular spiritual leader constitute a kind of "religious family" that may also be called upon as a significant source of social support and influence.

Adherents generally view the relationship between their own healing practices and Western medicine as complementary rather than competitive. While spiritual leaders believe in the efficacy of their own remedies, they often advise their patients to go to Western doctors as well. There is a general belief that Western medicine treats the symptom of the problem (i.e., the manifestation of illness), while religious rituals treat its cause (i.e., the spiritual imbalance). In some cases, spiritual healers may see their contributions as assisting and increasing the efficacy of a doctor's efforts (this is especially the case for invasive and technologically mediated procedures such as surgery that are viewed both as efficacious and dangerous).

DRESS & MODESTY

Generally, there is no specific religious garb that believers wear on a daily basis. Santería and Candomblé devotees may, however, wear distinctive bead necklaces and bracelets (including ankle bracelets), which act as both a distinctive badge of membership and spiritual protection. Patients may also choose to wear charms or amulets that are believed to ward off evil spirits.

The beads, bracelets, charms, and amulets should not be removed without the patient's consent. If these items must be removed, it is usually preferred that the bead necklaces and bracelets be removed only by the person wearing them and that they not be touched by anyone else. If the patient is unable either to remove them himself/herself or grant consent for their removal, medical personnel can remove them. They should be handled respectfully and placed in a secure location.

There is one instance during which both Santería and Candomblé require particular religious garb. During the period of a year or more following a novice's initiation into the priesthood, the person is expected to dress entirely in white clothes and to wear head coverings (a hat for men or a white cloth tied around their head for women). Women may wear long white dresses, coats, jackets, and stockings that cover most of their bodies. Both men and women in this situation are viewed as especially vulnerable, and white is seen as a spiritually pure color that protects that vulnerability. It is important that people in this situation continue to be dressed only in white clothes and be allowed some form of white head covering if at all possible.

PRAYER & RITUAL OBSERVANCES

It is difficult to give a generalized summary of the Afro-Caribbean rituals that might occur in a health care setting. Given the secrecy surrounding rituals, it is virtually impossible to give specific examples of what a health care provider might encounter, making it especially important to discuss religious needs with patients and their families.

The secrecy surrounding healing rituals also highlights patients' need for privacy. While adherents of other religions may best be served with a meditation/quiet room, the ritual and religious needs of Afro-Caribbean patients can often be better met by providing privacy in their own hospital room, thereby allowing community members to visit and perform rituals with discretion.

In almost every case, the first step in healing rituals is to determine the spiritual cause of the ailment. This determination itself is a ritual, and is likely to be followed by other rituals designed to address the underlying cause. This undertaking usually will have occurred before a patient chooses to access Western medical care. If the cause of the patient's illness has already been determined by the spiritual leader, there is no need to perform divination at the hospital or clinic, but a diviner may be called in if the patient needs their help in making a decision of some kind. Given the nature of the divination procedures, there is no reason they cannot be performed in private in a health care setting without comprising sterility or disturbing other patients.

Different healing ceremonies accompany different spiritual diagnoses. Two patients with identical Western medical diagnoses may perform drastically different rituals if the spiritual leader believes that the spiritual causes of the malady are different. While the rituals are likely to vary according to the country of origin and the particular religious tradition of the patient, some general guidelines are:

- The healing rituals most likely to occur in health care settings are those in which something must be done to, for, or with the patient in their immediate environment. These would include prayers, ritual baths, cleansings with flowers, candle burning, or rituals that involve applying lotions or oils to the body or a variety of plant substances to the head. Practitioners will need to work with patients and their families to understand these rituals and accommodate them insofar as they are possible in a hospital setting.

- Although the conditions of some patients are such that the prescribed healing ritual will require live animal sacrifices, it is highly unlikely such rituals will be attempted in a hospital or clinic setting. The objective in these sacrifices is to secure the animal's blood in order to apply it to icons of the deities, so that these sacrifices are most appropriately done in front of an altar.

- The major deities worshipped do not enter the bodies of their devotees and priests outside of religious ceremonies, so spirit possession is extremely unlikely to occur in a health care setting.

As part of their general spiritual observances, patients may bring in icons of saints, candles, or natural objects (e.g., rocks, sticks, etc). These should not be touched without patient consent. Patients' families may also bring food, so providers may need to discuss any applicable dietary restrictions with patients and their families.

HYGIENE & WASHING REQUIREMENTS

Hygiene and personal cleanliness are very important to most people from Afro-Caribbean traditions. It is important to provide patients with washing facilities, particularly postnatal women. Many patients will feel more comfortable with relatives assisting them in the cleansing process rather than health care providers.

In addition to regular bathing, a few patients might take ritual baths at the suggestion of their spiritual leaders. These baths are not typically all-water baths, but contain other substances, such as perfume, milk, honey, palm oil, wine, or leafy herbs. Some Afro-Caribbean patients may also wish to add an antiseptic to bath water. Typically, a spiritual leader will determine what substances should be added to the water based on his/her understanding of the causes of illness.

It is unlikely that a health care provider will be involved with this particular practice, because ritual baths typically occur in private residences where they are either self-administered or administered by a spiritual leader. If it does come up in a health care setting and a bath is not available (or not advisable), it is best to discuss alternatives with the patient such as providing a basin of water big enough so that the patient can stand in it. It may be useful for providers to ask whether patients have engaged in a ritual bath, especially in the case of a skin ailment or irritation. Practitioners may need to work with patients to understand what substances are being used and how these may be interacting with other treatments.

DIETARY REQUIREMENTS

Santería, Candomblé, Vodoun, and Palo Mayombe have no explicit, universal dietary restrictions.

Many Rastafarians eschew pork and salt and follow Jewish dietary laws as well as a modified vegan diet called *ital* (from the word "vital"). The general principle of ital is that food should be eaten in its natural state. Thus, some Rastafarians avoid food which is chemically modified or contains artificial additives (e.g., color and preservatives); strict interpretations prohibit foods produced using chemical pesticides and fertilizer. Most Rastafarians avoid all red meat, many do not eat fish (or at least fish that are over 12 inches in length, and some are strict vegetarians. Some also avoid shellfish.

Adherents of Afro-Christian churches also may ascribe healing properties to certain foods, and may wish to maintain a diet that they believe provides spiritual balance. These dietary restrictions exist in Santería, Candomblé, Vodoun, and Palo Mayombe and stem from one's relationships with the specific spirits or deities one serves. For example, in Santería, the orisha *Oshún* is believed to keep all her magic herbs and sacred objects inside a pumpkin; she is also associated with the patron saint of Cuba, La Virgen de la Caridad del Cobre. Therefore, those who worship Oshún are barred from eating pumpkins, which are a special food reserved for the orisha. This dietary restriction is especially important on Oshún's/La Virgen's Feast Day, which falls on September 8.

Many patients will prefer to eat food brought by friends and relatives. This should be accommodated if possible. If there are any medically indicated dietary restrictions, they should be explained to the patient and family.

MEDICATION, TREATMENT, AND PROCEDURE RESTRICTIONS

Generally, patients will not object to particular medications, treatments, or procedures. Most do not view the different methods of healing as competitive, but rather as mutually beneficial. However, they may wish to combine medication prescribed by a Western medical practitioner with herbal remedies prescribed by a traditional healer. In addition, patients may not offer information about the herbal remedies they are taking, so that it is useful to inquire.

Many Rastafarian patients will observe a series of dietary restrictions that can inform what medications they will or will not accept.

GENDER & MODESTY

Many patients prefer to be seen by a provider of the same sex due to cultural beliefs surrounding modesty; typically, these preferences are not religiously motivated.

ORGAN DONATION

Santería, Candomblé, Vodoun, and Palo Mayomblé have not taken any binding positions concerning organ donation. Although organ donation and reception are generally permissible, each patient should be consulted to determine his/her personal preferences.

Members of Afro-Christian churches may be expected to have fairly positive attitudes to organ donation and reception. The religio-political positions of Rastafarians and their suspicion of whites and white institutions may incline them to oppose donating or receiving organs but, once again, it is best to query the individual patient.

INFORMED CONSENT & PATIENT DECISION MAKING

Close bonds between immediate and extended family members is common in Afro-Caribbean culture. In Santería, Candomblé, and Vodoun, devotees led by the same spiritual leader often consider themselves a religious family and have a variety of quasi familial obligations to each other that may be very significant, especially for older patients who have outlived or are far away from biological relatives.

Patients will often want older and respected members of the family to be involved in health care decision making (and those who are very religious may want the advice of a diviner or spirit medium). Some may even expect bad news (e.g., poor prognoses) to be shared with the oldest immediate family member first.

In order to avoid possible conflict, the provider may wish to clarify with the patient and family early on in treatment that prognoses are given to the patient first, unless s/he explicitly requests otherwise. It may also be necessary to take the religious family into account in discharge planning because this group may be a significant part of the patient's support system.

REPRODUCTIVE HEALTH & FAMILY PLANNING

For many Afro-Caribbean women, there is strong social pressure to give birth. In most cases, the husband prefers to be included in discussions of contraception or sterilization. However, it is not unusual for women to make the decisions on contraception and family planning themselves.

Culturally, abortion is largely discouraged and is accompanied by a social stigma. However, there is quite a bit of knowledge of herbal abortifacients that circulates among women and is known to spiritual leaders.

When there are infertility problems, a couple might seek the advice of a religious leader who can diagnose the spiritual cause. Either a woman's or a man's actions might be blamed for reproductive problems, so this issue should be addressed with great sensitivity.

In Haitian Vodoun, there is a specific belief involving pregnant women called perdition (pedisyon) that may become an issue. It is believed that during pregnancy, the menstrual blood that normally exits during a woman's period is held in the womb as nourishment for the child. However, in a state of perdition, the nourishing blood bypasses the fetus, arresting the pregnancy. A fetus may stay in a state of arrested growth for years; when the child is able to "untie" itself from the state of perdition, the pregnancy resumes and childbirth follows. The most frequent cause of perdition is believed to be sorcery.

Providers discussing issues around menstruation or infertility with adherents of Haitian Vodoun should be aware that this may be an issue for patients. Sometimes, for example, patients with menstrual irregularities may delay seeking treatment, believing that they are in perdition.

PREGNANCY & BIRTH

Women may take special herbal remedies believed to aid in the health of the child during their pregnancies, so providers should inquire which, if any, herbs a pregnant patient is using. In addition, pregnant and postnatal women are thought to be especially vulnerable to supernaturally influenced health problems. Thus, many choose to stay inside and avoid strenuous activities.

There are rituals that accompany childbirth in each Afro-Caribbean religion. These generally are done at home several days to two weeks after the birth and are highly unlikely to occur inside a hospital. If the family needs to perform a ritual in a hospital setting, privacy should be given if possible.

Amulets or charms may be placed around the baby's wrist to ward off evil spirits.

It is common for mothers to have a great deal of support from older women in their families during childbirth. Traditionally, new mothers rest for anywhere from two weeks to 1½ months after childbirth. During this time, female relatives or neighbors help care for the mother and newborn.

In some Afro-Caribbean cultures, women believe that new mothers must avoid any activities that might cause a chill. For a few days after birth, the mother might therefore be reticent to wash her hair. Additionally, some women do not cook or handle certain foods while bleeding after birth. In other traditions, however, mothers may wish to bathe themselves frequently after giving birth. Caretakers should check with the new mother regarding her preferences.

END OF LIFE

Given the importance of extended family and faith communities, an Afro-Caribbean patient is likely to receive a large number of visitors if death appears to be imminent. Many will not be restrained in their expression of mourning. A space for visitors to congregate and privacy during these visits would be appreciated.

There are elaborate rituals in Afro-Caribbean religions surrounding death, many of which are not shared openly. One example that has been made public is the Haitian Vodoun death ritual. Practitioners of Haitian Vodoun believe that the dead body can be separated from the various spiritual entities that animate it. Haitian Vodoun teaches that each human has both a *gwo bonanj* (big guardian angel) and a *lwa* (spirit). Shortly after death, the gwo bonanj must be removed from the person through the death ritual. During this ritual, the dead also speak to the living through spirit possession; the spirits of the deceased often inquire about living family members, and raise problems that they are able to observe within the community.

This is only one of the many rituals that may take place post death. Most others are unknown to those who are not initiates of the particular traditions. Thus, it is important to work closely with members of both the biological and religious families to determine what actions health care providers need to take after a devotee, priest, or priestess has died. In this way, many costly and emotionally wrenching errors can be avoided.

FOR MORE READING: AFRO-CARIBBEAN TRADITIONS

Brandon GE. Healing in African and African-derived religions. In: Glazier S, ed. *Encyclopedia of African and African-American Religions.* New York, NY: Routledge. 2001: 132-139.

Brown KM. Afro-Caribbean spirituality: A Haitian case study. In: Sullivan LE, ed. *Healing and Restoring: Health and Medicine in the World's Religious Traditions.* New York, NY: Macmillan. 1989: 255-285.

Chavkin W, Busner C, McLaughlin M. Reproductive health: Caribbean women in New York City, 1980-1984. *Int Migr Rev.* 1987; 21[3]: 609-625.

Jones SG. The Caribbean/West Indies cultural competency program for Florida nurses implications for HIV/AIDS prevention and treatment. *J Multicult Nursing Health.* Winter 2005

Laguerre MS. *Afro-Caribbean Folk Medicine: The Reproduction & Practice of Healing.* S Hadley, MA: Bergin Garvey; 1988.

Sandoval MC. Santería: Afrocuba concepts of disease and its treatment in Miami. *J Oper Psychiatry.* 1977: 8[2]: 52-63.

Schott J, Henley A. Traditional Afro-Caribbean culture. In: Schott J, Henley A., eds. *Culture, Religion and Childbearing in a Multiracial Society.* Oxford, UK: Butterworth-Heinemann. 1996: 243-248.

PART IV

• • • •

Practitioners' Responsibilities

• • • •

Practitioners' Responsibilities

Six Steps to a Religiously Inclusive Practice

Organizational Resources

PART 4: PRACTITIONERS' RESPONSIBILITIES

1
••••
Practitioners' Responsibilities

As you saw in Section A, many patients bring religion along with them when they come for health care. This reality can create barriers-unless practitioners address religion and use what they learn to help their patients. When they do, there are real benefits to be had both for patients and practitioners. Practitioners skilled in addressing religion with patients build more open provider-patient relationships, which can reveal key information about patient behaviors and health-related beliefs. Not only does this help reduce culturally and religiously motivated barriers to health care, it also results in bottom-line benefits that benefit the providers themselves.

As our country's demographics change, practitioners are treating more and more diverse patient populations. The United States now has significant Muslim, Sikh, Hindu, and Buddhist populations. Increased immigration from Africa and the Caribbean is bringing syncretic traditions such as Voudon and Candomblé. Adherents of these traditions may have attitudes about health and illness or use traditional healing methods that are foreign to US-trained providers. Sometimes, these can create obstacles to care. There are instances where a community's religious and cultural issues are so significant that the community members refrain from accessing the health care they need and deserve. Ignoring these issues doesn't just compromise a single patient's care. It can result in disparate care of entire communities.

All of this means that practitioners today have a responsibility to become culturally and religiously competent in order to provide the best possible care. Being a competent provider amidst all this diversity requires that practitioners know how to navigate the diverse beliefs and practices of their current (and future) patients.

But this is a general statement. What are the particular responsibilities of different providers throughout the health care system? The answer is not that simple. While there are some particular responsibilities that doctors, nurses, social workers, and others might be expected to assume, more often than not, the appropriate role and scope of activity will depend on the specific situation.

The following, therefore, are general guidelines for health care professionals that set forth some of the responsibilities they can be expected to assume to provide religio-culturally competent care:

PART 4: PRACTITIONERS' RESPONSIBILITIES

PHYSICIANS

Depending on the length and intensity of a relationship, the frequency of contact, and the doctor's own comfort level, a doctor may have a more or less extensive role working with a patient's religious needs.

In general, it is important for doctors to effectively determine how religion may be affecting a patient's health care decisions including such issues as compliance with medication routines and the use of alternative remedies. They also may need to respond when patients raise the issue directly or indirectly. For example, a long-term patient may request to pray with the doctor, or may ask the doctor to be present during a religious ritual.

In addition, doctors are likely to periodically liaise with a patient's family, a pastoral care professional, or a clergyperson for assistance with particular issues (e.g., if the patient objects to certain treatments, wishes to follow specific dietary practices, or is incorporating traditional/alternative healing methods into his/her care).

NURSES AND NURSES' AIDES

Most nurses performing day-to-day care will need to know about modesty, diet, hygiene, and other basic religious requirements, and may be called on to assist patients with religious requirements including ritual cleansing, donning religious garments, or engaging in prayer. It can be a good idea for nurses to have relationships with pastoral care staff. Given the frequency with which nurses and aides interact with patients (especially hospitalized patients), they may be in the best position to become aware of unmet religious needs or spiritual distress and can assist with getting those needs met in an appropriate manner or in procuring a referral to pastoral care.

SOCIAL WORKERS AND PHYSICAL/OCCUPATIONAL THERAPISTS

All allied health professionals should also be aware of religious requirements that may effect or conflict with recommended therapies (e.g., daily prayer times or attitudes toward opposite-sex providers). Social workers and PT/OTs may need to work with patients and families to explore ways that religious rituals or needs can be met or modified to allow for maximum participation for the patient.

A social worker may need to work with a patient to help him/her reconnect with a religious community or help the patient access his/her own sources of strength, which, for many, includes religion or spirituality (of course, this is a delicate task and the social worker needs to be careful, in assessing the patient, to make sure that this is a real need and not one that others, including the social worker him or herself, read into an assessment of patient's needs and desires). It might also be useful for social workers to have a list of resources to which they can refer those patients who prefer more support from religious rather than secular sources.

Physical and Occupational Therapists may need to work with patients to enable them to participate in the religious rituals they choose to observe; this might include therapy to help a patient regain full ability to engage in a particular ritual (e.g., rehabilitating a Muslim patient to help her regain the ability to fully engage in the physical aspects of Muslim prayer) or working with a patient to reshape a ritual to fit new physical restrictions (e.g., helping a severely injured Muslim patient identify ways to pray by altering the physicality of prayer).

In both cases, social workers and PT/OTs may also want to consult with a patient's clergyperson or a pastoral care professional.

PART 4: PRACTITIONERS' RESPONSIBILITIES

CHAPLAINS

Chaplains often serve as counselors or clergypersons, and can be useful as resources for other health care practitioners, bringing religious issues to their attention and helping patients connect (or reconnect) with religious communities, where appropriate.

Chaplains can also play an important role for practitioners—many are trained as educators, and can be a valuable resource for training around a range of religious and cultural competency issues. (For more information, see Working Effectively with Chaplains and Working Effectively with Chaplains: Resources.)

FAMILY, FRIENDS, AND OTHER CARETAKERS

Family, friends, and other caretakers can have widely varied roles and responsibilities in patients' lives, and there may be a range of ways to involve them in meeting patients' religious needs. For example, if a visiting nurse is dropping by each day at noon to check on a patient's home chemotherapy infusion, why not also take 2 minutes to assist his limited-mobility Orthodox Jewish patient with required washing before noontime prayer? Perhaps a friend who takes the patient grocery shopping can schedule her visit at a time when the patient also needs to get to church, or a relative visiting a Sikh patient who brings food from the langar can take the time to help the patient brush his hair and re-tie his turban.

Above all, it is critical to remember a patient's religious or spiritual needs are almost never *solely* the domain of a clergyperson or chaplain. Religion integrates itself into countless facets of life and health care, and all practitioners have a responsibility to be attuned to how it affects the care they offer and to respond appropriately.

2
....

Six Steps to a Religiously Inclusive Practice

Religious competency may seem like an overwhelming goal—there are thousands of religious traditions in the United States, and no one person can know everything there is to know about all of them. Just the idea that religious competence might involve absorbing this entire body of knowledge can be enough to deter some people from pursuing it at all.

Luckily, no one expects health care practitioners to know *everything* about religion and culture. Being aware of the need for religious competence in the clinical encounter, learning about the ways religion intersects with health care, understanding what resources are available to you, and knowing when to ask key questions are the responsibility of health care practitioners—and the way to religious competence.

The following six steps will help you make the transition to a more religio-culturally competent practice.

1. Commitment

The first step seems simple but it is the foundation for all the others. The provider has to be committed to making religio-cultural competence an important part of his/her practice. Training, materials, and patient assessment tools do no good without a commitment to using them properly.

Often, physicians and providers are pressed for time with their patients, and it can seem impossible to add even one more issue into the short time available for the patient encounter. But when it comes to religious competency, the benefit outweighs the cost. A little time invested can reap tremendous results. Committing to religious competency as a core part of clinical encounters—making it a non-negotiable piece of conversations with patients—ensures that key issues are not overlooked and adds depth to the provider-patient relationship.

2. Training

Health care practitioners don't become who they are without years of education and hands-on training. Just as a patient wouldn't want to be examined by a provider with no training in medical diagnosis, most patients won't want to discuss religion (for many, an incredibly personal and sensitive topic) with a provider who is not trained to do so respectfully and effectively.

Training in religious competence—what to ask, how and when to ask it, and what to do with the information once you have it—is a critical step to becoming religiously competent. Starting a conversation about religion without understanding some basic communication guidelines can easily result in a highly uncomfortable experience for provider and patient alike.

Ideally, training should be provided to anyone who has direct contact with patients, from physicians to nurses to phlebotomists to visiting volunteers. They are all part of the health care team, and religion may be implicated in any one of their areas of expertise.

Read Section B: Understanding Your Patients for some communication dos and don'ts.

3. Assessments

Once you know what to ask and how to ask it, it's time to start putting these new skills into practice. Make religious and spiritual assessment part of your regular patient assessment process.

This will take different forms, depending on the setting. For providers working in solo or group practices who see the bulk of their patients for checkups and routine matters, a simple question or two about religious affiliation and significant practices around diet and dress may be enough. For providers working in a hospital or long-term care facility, a more in-depth conversation is probably warranted. (Use our checklist as a starting point!)

4. Resources

Commitment and training notwithstanding, every physician or provider is going to run up against unfamiliar beliefs or practices that influence a patient's treatment, compliance, or their experience of the health care system in an unexpected way. Knowing your resources and how to locate them quickly will make all the difference.

Tools like this manual are a great support, as are all the materials listed in the resources section. It's also helpful to maintain contact information for pastoral care professionals or community clergy from a wide variety of denominations (use our Chaplaincy Checklist to keep this information close at hand). Being prepared helps ensure that you'll be able to access the information you need in time-sensitive situations.

5. Patient Materials

The onus for religio-cultural competency does not fall solely on the provider—the patient also has a responsibility to disclose any religious beliefs or practices that might influence his/her reaction to treatment. But just as providers aren't always aware of the range of ways in which religious beliefs can influence health care, patients may not always know what information about their beliefs their providers need.

When patients understand that certain information about their religious needs may be useful to their providers, they become part of the process. Provide materials for patients (like a version of our checklist, adapted for patients) that explain what kinds of information are useful for a provider to have. A few pamphlets left in the waiting room and an informed patient can mean that the provider will spend less time getting to the root of the patient's medical issue.

6. Décor

Religious and cultural inclusivity should be reflected in surroundings as well as actions. In all likelihood, you serve patients from all religious, cultural, and ethnic backgrounds. All of those patients deserve to walk into a doctor's office or hospital and feel as though it is a place where they will receive quality, whole-person treatment.

When redecorating or arranging the office, work to ensure that the décor and materials in the space are welcoming to and reflective of a multicultural patient population. Holiday decorations, especially around December, should be kept religiously neutral (see Key Interventions: Negotiating the December Dilemma, for more on how to do this).

Becoming religiously and culturally competent doesn't have to be an overwhelming task, and you've already made the first move by accessing this manual. Breaking the process down into six manageable steps makes this important process clear and accessible.

3

Organizational Resources

PRACTITIONERS' ROLES & RESPONSIBILITIES: ORGANIZATIONAL RESOURCES

Keep copies of this checklist with other patient assessment materials.

As you learned in Section A, many patients bring religion with them when accessing health care, whether practitioners would prefer that they do so or not. But when practitioners learn to talk about religion and use what they learn to help their patients, rewards and opportunities abound: deeper provider-patient relationships, the opportunity to learn more about patient behaviors and health-related beliefs, and the ability to break down culturally and religiously motivated barriers to health care (along with some significant bottom-line benefits).

You may think that helping patients get their religious needs met is outside of your job description and is the chaplain's role, but there are often ways you can enhance the care you provide by being aware of important religious or cultural factors. Sometimes, providing the best possible care may mean you have a responsibility to pay attention to religious issues.

If you're having trouble determining whether a patient's religious needs implicate your role, it can be helpful to ask yourself what your precise medical responsibilities vis-à-vis this patient are. For example, are any of the following implicated:

- Diet or nutrition issues;

- Extended hospital stays or outpatient visits of more than minimal duration;

- Prescription medications;

- Surgical procedures, whether major or minor;

- Sexual and reproductive health; and/or

- Severe or terminal illness?

PART 4: PRACTITIONERS' RESPONSIBILITIES

Each of these areas commonly implicates religious concerns, which can have a significant impact on patient decision making. You may also want to ask yourself the following:

- What is my connection with this patient? Is it a one-time encounter, or an ongoing relationship?

- Have I ever spoken with this patient about religious needs?

- (If the patient is hospitalized) Do I know whether pastoral care has visited this patient? If so, have I connected with the relevant chaplain?

PART V

••••

Key Interventions

••••

Setting Boundaries: Proselytizing & Inappropriate Religious Expression in a Health Care Setting

Working with Family, Friends, and Other Caregivers

Working Effectively with Chaplains

Pastoral Care Resources

Navigating the December Dilemma

Overcoming Barriers to Care

1

Setting Boundaries: Proselytizing & Inappropriate Religious Expression in a Health Care Setting

At the end of a training session on religious competency in health care, the facilitator asked all the participants to list one thing they had learned that they planned to incorporate into their practices. One woman, a nurse, proudly replied that she would no longer turn on televised Christian worship services every Sunday morning for all her patients, nor would she offer blessings to all of them.

This woman may have been an excellent nurse, and her actions may have been motivated by the best of intentions — to encourage religious or spiritual behaviors as an aid in healing, to offer comfort, or to help her patients find salvation. But well-meaning or not, her conduct was inappropriate and may have had a real negative impact on the patients for whom she cared.

Proselytizing and other inappropriate religious expressions are problematic in health care settings, where people are ill, health care providers are those who deliver the needed care *as well as* comfort, and there is a power differential between patient and practitioner. Inappropriate religious expression can corrode the patient-provider relationship, creating mistrust and leading to poor communication. Even when the provider's personal experience is that spirituality improves the chances of a good outcome in times of illness, it is up to the provider to listen carefully to the patient and avoid raising issues that the patient does not welcome or request.

The strict definition of proselytizing is what occurs when one person attempts to convince another of the correctness of his/her religious beliefs. In some religions, such as evangelical Christianity, Mormonism, and the Jehovah's Witness tradition, among others, conversion is actually a religious duty, viewed as an act of kindness toward the person to be converted.

"Inappropriate religious expression," is the term used in this manual. It covers proselytizing but also refers to the broader range of communications that do not necessarily rise to that level (i.e., communications that do not overtly attempt to convert), but still cross a line or can be unwelcome or offensive to the person at whom it is directed. Examples include:

- Praying over or reciting a blessing for someone who has not requested that you do so;

- Asking someone who has not indicated an interest in discussing religion whether or not s/he is "saved";

- Bringing a religious item or text to someone who has not requested that you do so;

- Encouraging someone to pray, meditate, attend worship service, or otherwise engage in religious or spiritual activities for the good of their health; and

- Inviting someone whose religious affiliation and comfort level you don't know to attend a worship service, prayer group, or scriptural study.

Even expression that may seem completely innocuous, such as signing off an email or phone message with a blessing, may be unwelcome and can cause problems.

As with the nurse mentioned above, such communiqués can create discomfort, though they often stem from a desire to provide reassurance and strength in a time of stress. Published studies claiming to document a positive correlation between religion or spiritual behaviors and health outcomes may also encourage some providers to cross the line and promote such beliefs and behaviors as aids to healing. Proselytizing also often becomes an issue at the end of life, when the provider may be concerned not just for the patient's comfort, but for his/her soul or sense of peace.

However, unlike a co-worker or acquaintance with whom you might be on equal footing, the practitioner-provider relationship involves an unequal power dynamic. The patient has a problem and is dependent on the practitioner to solve it. When a physician or provider proselytizes or talks about religion in an inappropriate way, the patient may feel that s/he is being judged or coerced, or worry about whether s/he will receive the best care if s/he does not follow what the provider believes.

This can destroy the trust on which the practitioner-patient relationship is based: it can make the patient feel as though the physician or provider is attempting to impose his/her agenda rather than offer the best possible care (even if the provider *is* offering the best possible care). With a patient already under the stress of dealing with a medical issue, this concern can become an additional obstacle to healing.

There are several steps you can take to minimize inappropriate religious expression, whether you are a solo provider or a practitioner working in a large facility:

- *Pay attention to your own communications.* Remember you are in a position of authority, and that your words can carry extra weight. If your religion calls on you to proselytize, you should follow that doctrine according to your belief while being mindful of your duties and responsibilities as a provider of quality, patient-centered health care which means — *not* proselytizing at work.

- *Learn more about respectful and cross-cultural communication,* and practice those skills.

PART 5: KEY INTERVENTIONS

- *Speak up.* If you think a colleague may be sharing too much about his/her faith, approach him/her gently and ask him/her to reconsider the conduct; if that has no result, approach a supervisor. If you see behavior you consider truly egregious, it is to the benefit of the patient to bring it up.

- If you are in a position to support professional development efforts or influence policy, do what you can to ensure that the providers with whom you work are trained in the boundaries of acceptable communication. Having clear policies around expression backs up your commitment to a facility free of proselytizing.

There may be circumstances in which a patient *asks* a provider to pray with (or for) him/her. In these situations, the response depends on the comfort level of the particular provider. If a provider is uncomfortable, s/he might offer to find another provider of the patient's religious tradition or a pastoral care professional to pray with the patient. A provider may also choose to remain with the patient while the patient prays, offering his/her presence while abstaining from prayer.

In some instances, there can also be a kind of "reverse" or anti-religion proselytizing—situations where practitioners attempt to *dissuade* patients of their religious beliefs or impose their own belief in the efficacy of a certain course of treatment. This can be just as problematic as traditional proselytizing.

Consider a few examples:

> An otherwise healthy woman visits her physician for a preoperative checkup; she is about to enter the hospital for a minor surgical procedure. At the end of the appointment, the doctor asks whether she has any additional concerns. She explains that she is confident all would go well, but that she would like a Catholic priest called in to administer Last Rites should anything happen. In an apparent attempt to reassure her, the physician responds, "Oh please, you don't really believe that stuff, do you?" She chooses another surgeon, not trusting her first surgeon to carry out her wishes if necessary.

> An older man with Parkinson's disease calls his neurologist with a question: Yom Kippur is approaching, and he plans to fast. For him, that means abstaining from ingesting anything, including his Parkinson's medication and the liquid required to swallow it. His condition is such that skipping the medication would not have a long-term detrimental effect, but would probably compromise his motor skills temporarily. The physician doesn't explain this and simply tells the patient to take the medication as directed.

In both of these cases, the practitioner opted to impose his/her own beliefs about the relative importance of religion over the patient's beliefs and religious needs—when there was no medical necessity to do so. An important part of the patient's identity was ignored, and a valuable opportunity to deepen (or to sustain) the physician-patient relationship was lost.

Effective and patient-centered care always requires that the practitioner be aware of his/her own beliefs and avoid imposing them on the patient, whether through overt proselytizing, well-intentioned prayer or blessing, uninvited encouragement to become more spiritual, or "reverse" proselytizing. Understanding and being aware of one's own religious and cultural lens is the first step to true religio-cultural competence.

2
....
Working with Family, Friends, & Other Caregivers

In many cases, especially when working with patients who are elderly, very young, or have long-term or degenerative conditions, practitioners must work closely with other caregivers including family members, friends, visiting or live-in nurses, or other allied health professionals. These individuals can be tremendous assets in helping a patient get all of his/her religious needs met.

When working with family, friends, and other caregivers, there are three broad issues to think through:

1. What do these other caregivers need to know about the patient's religious background and needs?

2. In what ways can these other caregivers be most helpful in getting those religious needs met?

3. What impact will the caregiver's own religious and cultural background have on the relationship?

Thinking through each of these while planning a patient's discharge, home care, or long-term hospital stay can help the practitioner create an effective and comprehensive team.

1. What do caregivers need to know?
In all situations, regardless of how circumscribed the caretaker's role is, s/he will most likely need to know certain basics: whether the patient has any religious beliefs related to modesty and gender, whether there is any religious figure the patient will want to speak with before consenting to a particular treatment, and significant holy days on which there are special observances and how the patient actually prefers to observe them.

Modesty issues often inform the way a person relates to people of the opposite sex or the topics they are willing to discuss with caretakers, while informed consent is a potential issue in almost any health care encounter. Holy days often come with celebrations, prescribed rituals, fasting or special foods, and worship services, all things that have an impact on a patient's daily life. Whether the caregiver is the child of an elderly patient or a once-a-week occupational therapist, there is the potential for each of these issues to arise.

Depending on the severity of the patient's condition and the caregiver's role, however, there can be a much wider range of knowledge needed:

> *A live-in nurse or family member* will likely need to know about a full range of issues: dietary requirements, dress and modesty requirements, prayer and ritual observances, and any restrictions on particular medications and procedures. S/He will need to know about any religious objects that might be encountered in the home and how these items should be handled, if at all. If the patient is terminal or in a hospice situation, the nurse or family member will need to know about the patient's religious views on palliative care and end-of-life/post death rituals. A caretaker with this level of involvement will also want to have contact information for the patient's clergyperson or religious community (if applicable).
>
> *Caretakers with more specialized roles* will obviously require less information to perform their duties effectively. A nonreligious family member who undertakes to prepare food for an observant Muslim grandparent may need to be informed of the precise halal requirements. A friend who visits daily to spend time with the patient will need to know if there are any designated prayer times during the day so that the friend can either visit at different times or, alternatively, schedule the visit during prayer time in order to provide needed assistance. A physical therapist working with a patient with limited mobility will need to know about religious rituals the patient may wish to be able to perform.

When working with these alternate caregivers, think carefully about the nature of their role in the patient's life and the potential ways they might interact with the patient. Use that analysis when deciding what information should be shared.

2. Where can the caregiver be most helpful?

Once the caregiver's role is understood and the relevant information shared, the next step is to determine whether there are other ways in which s/he could be helpful in getting the patients' religious needs met.

If a visiting nurse is dropping by each day at noon to check on a patient's home chemotherapy infusion, could s/he also take 2 minutes to assist the limited-mobility Orthodox Jewish patient with required washing before noontime prayer? Perhaps a friend who takes the patient grocery shopping can schedule the visit at a time when the patient also needs to get to church, or a relative visiting a Sikh patient who brings food from the langar can help the patient brush his hair and re-tie his turban.

Many observant religious people have a variety of religious practices, rituals, and prohibitions that influence virtually every facet of their everyday lives. Helping a patient in need of ongoing care to get all these needs met can seem like a daunting task. By taking advantage of a patient's network of extended caregivers and thinking creatively about how they may be helpful, this tremendous task is pared down to a manageable size.

3. What impact will the caregiver's own religious and cultural background have on the patient relationship?

Becoming religiously competent in patient interactions is itself a challenge, made even more difficult when a long-term care situation with multiple caregivers throws many personalities into the mix.

Although the care that family, friends, and other caregivers can provide is invaluable, there may be issues that arise when the caregiver has different beliefs from the patient—whether s/he is of another faith, is a nonbeliever or is dismissive of the patient's religious commitments.

Caregivers from other religious traditions often lack relevant knowledge and may need more careful explanations of (and training in) particular practices of other traditions. For example, if a Christian provider is working with an Orthodox Jew, it is useful for him to know that many observant Orthodox Jews will not eat food produced in a non-kosher kitchen, even if the ingredients themselves are kosher. Less observant Jews may eat food from a non-kosher kitchen, but not if the food came in contact with a prohibited food; furthermore, a utensil used to handle a non-kosher food and then dipped into a kosher one can render the food impermissible. Although many people understand that being kosher bars pork or the mixing of milk and meat, the particulars of these requirements are also significant. Understanding them allows the caregiver to know what to ask the patient to ensure that care responds to the person's needs.

Learning such information can be helpful in other situations. What about an art therapist working with an observant Muslim woman who has a conflict and asks a male colleague to cover for her, only to learn that the woman will not allow a man into her home when her husband is out? Or an aide who comes to help a patient with bathing and showering and leaves the patient's religious garments in a ball on the floor, seriously disturbing the patient?

Like providers, caregivers may also bring their own faiths into the patient relationship. The proselytizing and inappropriate religious expression that can be so problematic in a health care relationship with a provider also appear in some patient relationships with nonphysician caregivers, and the same power dynamic may be at play (although it may be somewhat lessened). Thus, for example, if the transportation aide who helps a patient run errands is a Jehovah's Witness and leaves a copy of *The Watchtower* behind, the patient may feel offended or uncomfortable but may not want to risk speaking up lest she lose her sole form of transportation.

The value that family, friends, and other caregivers provide is priceless, both to the patient and his/her regular practitioner. Taking the time to understand the patient's needs and devoting some careful thought to the abilities and skills provided by his/her caretakers can bring care to the next level, not only caring for physical issues but helping the patient become his/her full self.

PART 5: KEY INTERVENTIONS

3

Working Effectively with Chaplains

Even physicians and providers who fully appreciate the need for religio-cultural competence in patient care may be concerned about putting it into practice. There are certainly training programs and resources available (such as this one), but there are also many competing demands and a dearth of time in which to access them all. Often, religious and cultural issues are pushed to the side for the sake of medical expediency. For those practitioners working in hospitals or long-term care and rehabilitation facilities, there is a valuable—and often underused—resource that can make this process easier: the chaplain.

Chaplains and pastoral care departments can be found in most hospitals and large treatment facilities. However, they are often marginalized or underused because other practitioners may not know the breadth of their role. Understanding what a professional chaplain can bring to the table and making that chaplain a real part of the treatment team instantly brings a wealth of additional knowledge to bear on patient care.

For this to happen, practitioners need to:

1. Understand the role and skill-sets of a professional chaplain;

2. Examine the barriers that keep chaplains from becoming full members of the patient-care team in many facilities; and

3. Be aware of the range of ways in which chaplains can enhance patient care.

By making use of this valuable resource, practitioners can improve the quality of care offered and grow in their own religio-cultural competence.

WHAT CHAPLAINS ARE—AND WHAT THEY'RE NOT

Some of the failure to fully utilize pastoral care staff stems from a lack of understanding about who chaplains are and what they can offer.

Chaplains are not simply clergy people from the community (although they can be) or priests brought in to pray with dying patients (although they can be). They are not there only to pray with patients and certainly not to convert them; nor are they there to interfere with the medical care the physician determines is most appropriate for the patient.

Professional chaplains are highly trained clinical professionals who must log 600 hours of clinical education in addition to their theological education in order to be accredited. Their training includes intensive education in communication skills and patient assessment, as well as medical training to familiarize them with the types of illnesses and procedures they will see in a hospital setting. The Association of Professional Chaplains maintains standards of conduct and requirements, including ongoing pastoral and medical education.

All this prepares the professional chaplain to become meaningful partners in the patient care team, offering their clinical expertise alongside the physician, nurse, social worker, and other providers. Although a major part of the chaplain's role is helping patients whom illness has thrown into spiritual distress, chaplains can also operate much more broadly. Chaplains are professional caregivers prepared to work with all patients to enhance health and healing, regardless of faith or lack of faith.

Their skills in communication and spiritual assessment can help uncover additional relevant information about a patient. If there is a religious question about whether a patient can accept a certain treatment, a chaplain can mediate. If there is a religious practice that the patient is following that is causing harm, the chaplain can intervene. And chaplains bring a competency in the language of suffering and distress that can help patients better respond to his/her illnesses and find the strength to move through them.

Using chaplains effectively adds another layer to the patient treatment team and takes some pressure off the other practitioners. And because they bring a unique set of skills, the experience can be enriching for both patient *and* practitioner.

WHAT ARE THE BARRIERS TO EFFECTIVE USE OF CHAPLAINS?

There are a variety of reasons chaplains may not be used as well as they could be, some stemming from the physician or other provider, some from the chaplain, and some from institutional constraints as a whole:

- *Myths and stereotypes.* Many physicians and chaplains simply lack experience working with one another, leading to misperceptions about appropriate roles. A chaplain may assume that the physician will not be welcoming to the chaplain as part of the treatment team, while the physician may assume that the chaplain will proselytize the patient or should be called only if the patient needs to pray.

- *Discomfort around religion.* Often, chaplains are called in to work with patients who have already indicated a religious need or spiritual distress. However, patients with genuine religious needs sometimes go unnoticed because non-chaplaincy providers are not equipped or comfortable asking about religion and fail to take note of the patient's needs for a chaplain.

- *Secrecy.* Some chaplains are cautious about being openly religious in the more scientific milieu of a health care setting and therefore conduct their work in private; this can result in an effective, hard-working chaplain—and the results of his/her efforts—being invisible.

- *Interference with care.* Practitioners who don't understand what professional chaplains can bring to the table may be concerned that the chaplain will bring his/her religious views to bear on the situation to the detriment of a patient's medical needs, thereby interfering with treatment (e.g., by convincing the patient to reject a particular medication or procedure on religious grounds).

- *Religious bias.* Occasionally, providers who have had a bad experience with organized religion in the past will be hesitant or unwilling to call on pastoral care.

- *Insufficient resources.* In many health care settings, there are too few chaplains compared with the number of patients being served or chaplains who are not professionally trained. This can make it much more difficult to fully utilize the chaplains or to meet all the needs of the patients for chaplaincy services.

Most (if not all) of the barriers can be overcome, if one is willing to address the issue and some thoughtful education is provided on both religious competence and the roles and capabilities of pastoral care staff.

HOW TO USE CHAPLAINS

As noted above, chaplains are not simply people who pray with patients. They bring a range of skills and can be utilized in a variety of ways. The three broad ways in which chaplains can enhance the patient's experience and assist the other practitioners are:

1. As part of the treatment team;

2. As independent resources; and

3. As educators.

First, chaplains can be integral parts of the treatment team. They can and should participate in the initial patient assessment, as well as any reassessment that occurs if and when a patient's circumstances change. They can act as mediators between medical practitioners and family members, help patients maintain their links with their faith communities, and work within the health care facility to get the patient's religious needs met.

In their conversations with patients, chaplains can learn valuable information about the patient's religious, social, and cultural context that may inform treatment or even help with diagnosis. In addition, if a patient has a conflict between a religious belief or practice and a physician's proposed treatment, the chaplains can work with both parties to help them reach a mutually acceptable plan of action.

Importantly, chaplains also help patients access their personal sources of strength and comfort as they go through an illness or hospitalization. In so doing, they encourage patients to maintain the kind of positive attitude and coping skills that can help them to heal.

Second, chaplains are fantastic resources for issues of religious and cultural competency. Just as this Manual is a valuable, go-to resource for information, so are the chaplains in your institutions. A professional chaplain of any denomination can lend guidance on communication skills and how to have conversations around religious needs. Chaplains of particular denominations can provide more detailed information on that tradition's specific beliefs and practices.

Finally, chaplains can also serve as educators and advocates. The HealthCare Chaplaincy, one of the major pastoral education organizations in the New York Metro area, trains chaplains to serve not just individual patients, but the institutions in which they work. They are trained to be educators on religio-cultural competency and on conducting spiritual assessments for their institutions, and can be advocates pressing for more extensive cultural competency initiatives.

Chaplains add great value to patient-care teams as supports for the patient; as intermediaries among the patient, family, and physician; and as resources for religious or cultural issues. Learning to incorporate them fully into the team and to use them effectively improves the patient care experience for everyone involved.

4

Pastoral Care Resources

RESOURCES: CHAPLAINCY ORGANIZATIONS:

The HealthCare Chaplaincy
http://www.healthcarechaplaincy.org/
The HealthCare Chaplaincy is one of the largest multifaith, nonprofit centers for pastoral care, education, research, and consulting in the world. The Chaplaincy's clinical staff is intensively trained to provide professional spiritual care to patients, families, and staff of all faiths in numerous health care institutions throughout the greater New York region. Its accredited education programs teach clergy and qualified laypersons of all religious traditions the art and science of pastoral care.

In addition, its research and consulting services study best practices and promote quality assurance in pastoral care. The HealthCare Chaplaincy's Consulting Service offers a full range of options to institutions to begin or expand an existing pastoral care department.

The Association of Professional Chaplains
http://www.professionalchaplains.org/
The Association of Professional Chaplains (APC) serves chaplains in all types of health and human service settings. Its 4,000 members are chaplains involved in pastoral care, representing more than 150 faith groups. The APC advocates for quality spiritual care

PART 5: KEY INTERVENTIONS

of all persons in health care facilities, correctional institutions, long-term care units, rehabilitation centers, hospice, the military, and other specialized settings.

In addition, the APC offers continuing education courses and promulgates a code of conduct for professional chaplains.

RESOURCES: THE PHYSICIAN-CHAPLAIN RELATIONSHIP:

George Washington Institute for Spirituality and Health
Walking Together: Physicians, Chaplains, and Clergy Caring for the Sick,
http://www.gwish.org.cnchost.com/id81.htm (order form for booklet)

Vandecreek, Larry. *The Physician-Chaplain Relationship*.
Available for purchase through Amazon.com or local bookstores

Holst, Lawrence, ed. *Hospital Ministry: The Role of the Chaplain Today*.
Available for purchase through Amazon.com or local bookstores

5
....

Navigating the December Dilemma

The "December dilemma" is the time of year when multiple joyous religious holidays collide, and when people with good intentions can find themselves in the middle of potentially toxic misunderstandings and intolerance. The phenomenon occurs in institutions across America, from schools to hospitals.

In health care facilities, where people are coming to seek care and comfort, it is especially important to ensure that everyone who enters feels included. Depending on the demographic makeup of your staff and patient populations, real tensions could arise; Christian nurses working in a Jewish residential care facility may be cheered by Christmas decorations, but their patients and the patients' families probably don't feel the same way.

Although there are a range of religious holidays that can fall in December, there are five celebrations of which everyone should be aware. Keep these days in mind as you are scheduling staff or meetings, deciding on winter decorations for your facilities, or working out treatment and menu plans for the month of December:

> **1. Hanukkah**
> Hanukkah, also known as the Festival of Lights or Festival of Rededication, is an eight-day Jewish holiday that starts on the 25th day of Kislev, which may be in December, late November, or, more rarely, early January. The festival is observed in Jewish homes by lighting candles on each of the festival's eight nights, one on the first night, two on the second night, and so on. Prayers are recited during this ritual. In some families, Hanukkah also includes gift-giving.

2. Christmas Day

Christmas is a holiday celebrating the birth of Jesus, the central figure of Christianity. Aspects of the celebration may include gift-giving, Christmas trees, church attendance, the Father Christmas/Santa Claus myth, and family gatherings. Most Western churches (e.g., the Protestant and Roman Catholic traditions) observe the holiday on December 25, while most Eastern Orthodox Churches celebrate on January 7.

The one exception is Jehovah's Witnesses, who, although Christian, do not celebrate Christmas, believing that it has pagan roots (along with other holidays like Easter and Thanksgiving).

3. Kwanzaa

Kwanzaa (or *Kwaanza*) is a week-long secular holiday honoring African-American heritage and community, celebrated almost exclusively by African-Americans. It is observed from December 26 to January 1.

Kwanzaa consists of seven days of celebration, featuring activities such as candle lighting, drumming, and the pouring of libations, and culminates in a feast and gift-giving. It was founded by controversial black nationalist Ron Karenga in 1966 as a way to foster African-American unity and culture.

4. Bodhi Day

Bodhi Day is usually observed on December 8, or the Sunday immediately preceding. This is the date, according to Mahayana Buddhist tradition, of Siddhartha Gautama (the historical Buddha)'s Enlightenment and the beginning of his Buddhist teachings.

Bodhi Day is usually observed with prayer and meditation.

5. Ramadan

For more than a billion Muslims around the world—including the approximately 6 million in North America—Ramadan is a month of prayer, fasting, and charity. Muslims believe that during the month of Ramadan, Allah revealed the first verses of the Qur'an, the holy book of Islam. It often falls during November, December, or January.

Muslims practice sawm, or fasting, for the entire month of Ramadan. This means that they may not eat or drink anything, including water, during daylight hours. Ramadan ends with the festival of Eid al-Fitr, literally the "Festival of Breaking the Fast," which is one of the two most important Islamic celebrations. On Eid al-Fitr, people dress in their finest clothes, decorate their homes with lights and decorations, give treats to children, and enjoy visits with friends and family.

Acknowledging all these special occasions needn't be a difficult balancing act. By doing some careful thinking and using these guidelines as your roadmap, you can create a plan for dealing with the December dilemma that appreciates and addresses everyone's needs without sacrificing the festivity of the winter holidays.

Share the Wealth

Staff and colleagues can't address the December dilemma if they don't know about it. Distribute the Five to Know handout and educate staff on the types of holiday decorations and practices they might see in December. Consider a targeted training session to discuss the needs of the particular communities you serve and to formulate an action plan.

Pay Attention to Demographics

Understand both your staff/colleague and patient populations. They may not always be the same, and the types of celebrations or observances your staff may have in mind might not be what is most helpful for patients. Take a look at the demographics of these populations and try to anticipate both what staff will want (e.g., a menorah) with what will be most inclusive of your patient population (e.g., a non-denominational winter display).

Bear in mind that, as with proselytizing and religious expression, there is a power differential between providers and patients. In a hospital setting, providers get to go home at the ends of their shifts, but patients are stuck where they are. If holiday decorations or observances are offensive or exclusive, patients may feel this quite acutely.

Leverage Internal Diversity

Ask a diverse group of employees to plan holiday celebrations and/or displays to ensure that multiple voices and viewpoints are heard. Starting with diverse inputs is more likely to produce diverse, inclusive outputs.

Take Objections Seriously

Religion is a core part of personal identity for many people, and affronts to an individual's religion—whether real or perceived—can have a tremendous impact. In the case of provider-patient interactions, a problematic action does not simply cause offense; it also erodes the practitioner-patient relationship. If patients object to a particular holiday décoration or observance in your office, take those objections seriously.

The same goes for employees and colleagues: if someone raises an objection to a plan, activity, or decoration, take it seriously and act in the spirit of accommodation—just because a particular activity is traditional or seems innocuous doesn't mean it can't be cause for exclusion.

Honor Differences

Use appropriate greetings for your patients and colleagues. Stores have cards for Hanukkah and Kwanzaa, for example. Going this extra step sends an important message to your colleagues and patients that you value them as whole people.

Schedule Sensitively

For staff and colleagues, examine schedules so that vacations and personal days are spread among many, not a few. Staff responsible for scheduling patient appointments should also keep significant holiday dates in mind; a Jew may not want to come in on the first night of Hanukkah, nor may a Muslim want to fast for a blood test on the Eid.

By educating yourself and your colleagues and being mindful of a few straightforward guidelines, you can navigate the December dilemma with grace and respect.

6

Overcoming Barriers to Care

Some religious traditions — most notably, Christianity — are well known in the United States, and many people have a sense of their beliefs, practices, and holidays. Others, however, are little known; the result is that members of minority or marginalized religious communities may face barriers to care or find themselves otherwise alienated from mainstream health care systems.

Barriers to care are those religious and cultural issues that are so significant that they can keep entire populations from accessing the health care they need and deserve. Ignoring these issues doesn't just compromise a single patient's care, but can compromise an entire community's.

Consider a few examples:

- A Hmong woman was given a diagnosis of brain stem herniation, the only treatment for which is drilling holes in the skull to alleviate intercranial pressure. Her husband, the decision maker in Hmong culture, was reluctant to allow the surgery because one of the woman's souls was thought to be lost; Hmong believe that each person has multiple souls, and the woman's husband thought that if her soul were recovered she might heal, making surgery unnecessary.

    Doctors pressed for the surgery, and the husband became more and more resistant. He was ready to leave the hospital altogether, taking his seriously ill wife with him.

- Jehovah's Witnesses reject all blood products, including plasma/platelets. As many health care practitioners know, this often means that they will reject necessary surgical procedures that would result in blood loss and necessitate a transfusion. Jehovah's Witness parents will sometimes also reject these procedures for their children.

Many providers are frustrated by what they see as the patient's refusal to accept standard treatment. In each of these three cases, there is a significant barrier rendering care inaccessible—and the quality of care makes no difference if it is inaccessible to the patient, whether for language, mobility, cultural, or religious reasons. However, each of these cases also has a solution, arrived at by some creative thinking and the willingness to explore new alternatives, and the solutions carry benefits beyond the original issue.

In the case of the Muslim women rejecting the gowns, the facility took their concerns seriously and went back to the drawing board. Continuing to work with the community, the hospital developed a gown alternative: a flowing top and long, loose pants. The top and pants were loose enough to give physicians access to the patient, but provided enough coverage to satisfy the women.

The facility noticed an immediate and lasting increase in the number of Muslim women coming in for care. The hospital's proactive approach made health care accessible for this population, and the hospital earned a reputation in the community as a facility willing to reach out and make changes to broaden access for marginalized populations. The result? Loyal patients as well as improved health care for them.

For the seriously ill Hmong patient, the barrier was removed by a single sensitive physician. This physician entered the conversation and insisted that the family be allowed to connect with their own spiritual needs. The family went home and performed a ceremony to lure the woman's lost soul home. When she failed to recover after the ceremony, they brought her back to the hospital for surgery, after which she made a full recovery.

The husband had not disagreed with the surgery diagnosis, but was afraid that his wife would not survive surgery with a missing soul. Recognizing the family's desire to pursue their spiritual needs actually encouraged them to return to the hospital.

There are a variety of inventive new options now available to get around the Jehovah's Witness prohibition on blood and blood products. "Bloodless" procedures allow the patient to become their own blood bank by conserving blood (e.g., with medications that constrict arterial blood flow), recycling blood (e.g., by using "cell savers" that function like dialysis machines, re-infusing the patient's own blood), and through medications like Procrit that push a patient's bone marrow to produce more blood.

These procedures have the dual benefit of addressing Jehovah's Witness religious needs and addressing international blood shortage, matching, and safety issues. Currently, there are over 80 medical centers around the world where bloodless medicine and surgery are performed. Jehovah's Witnesses can be proud of the fact that they have been instrumental in causing bloodless surgery and other non-blood therapy to become viable alternatives, not only for Jehovah's Witnesses, but for the benefit of others as well.

If you are working with a person who is a Jehovah's Witness and don't have access to these options, it may be possible to find a facility to serve the patient that does. But if that is not possible and there is a life-saving emergency involving a young child, then the balancing between the parents' religious beliefs and the life of the child may require a different approach, including a consultation with legal counsel. (Hospitals may also seek court-ordered treatment for young children.)

Hopefully, your practice or institution is aware of the communities surrounding your facilities. Pay attention to which communities are accessing care routinely — preventative as well as emergency care — and which are not (if any). Is there a discrepancy between the groups you hope to serve and those you're actually serving? If so, there may be a religious or cultural barrier making your services inaccessible.

This barrier need not be insurmountable. Like the stories above, creative thinking and flexibility can help make your services accessible to all. Issues at play may include:

- *Dress*, as with the Muslim women above. Do you serve communities with modest dress requirements? Do your exam garments meet them?

- *Gender*. Do you serve communities in which people must see providers of the same sex? Is staff scheduled to ensure that your facility has a mixture of male and female physicians, nurses, and nurses' aides available?

- *Hours of operation*. Do you serve communities with religious observances that restrict when they can visit? For example, if you serve a large Orthodox Jewish community, do you have visitation hours late on Saturdays so that people with non-emergency issues can come in after the Sabbath has ended?

- *Traditional remedies*. Are you prepared to allow patients to use traditional or alternative remedies along with what you prescribe? Are the communities you serve aware of your openness?

Of course, this is not an exhaustive list of issues. To truly discover why a particular group is not accessing available health care, a facility will need to investigate, reaching out to the community to understand the reason and, if there is a problem, to understand its scope. Once that scope is determined, however, there is almost always a solution that opens health care to all.

ADDENDUM

• • • •

Checklists, Tools, & Organizational Resources

• • • •

Setting Boundaries

Navigating the December Dilemma

Working with Family, Friends, and Other Caregivers

Pastoral Care

Special Community Needs

ADDENDUM: CHECKLISTS, TOOLS, & ORGANIZATIONAL RESOURCES

1
....

Setting Boundaries: Organizational Resources

Ask Yourself: Am I Engaging in Appropriate Religious Self-expression? Keep copies of this checklist with other patient assessment materials.

1. Do I respect that other people's religions may differ from my own or that they may not believe in religion at all?

2. Am I sensitive to when and how I share my religious beliefs with others?

3. Am I careful to balance my personal religious expression (religious dress, jewelry, or objects) with its impact on others who may not share my faith (opening meetings with prayer or including religious language in company emails)?

4. Do I initiate prayer with colleagues or patients without being sure if those prayers are welcomed?

5. Am I doing my part to help maintain an inclusive environment in my workplace?

ADDENDUM: CHECKLISTS, TOOLS, & ORGANIZATIONAL RESOURCES

2

Navigating the December Dilemma

We've developed a checklist of actions that can help to create an inclusive environment during the holiday season. What will you try? Keep copies of this checklist with other patient assessment materials.

- ☐ **The Roundtable:** Ask a diverse group of co-workers to plan any holiday celebrations.

- ☐ **Be Curious:** Don't ignore questions. Encourage respectful curiosity.

- ☐ **Study! Study! Study!:** Review your facility's religion in the workplace policies to be clear on what is acceptable and not acceptable at December holiday time-and make no exceptions, especially in patient interactions.

- ☐ **Plan Your Work:** Examine schedules so that vacations and personal days are spread among many, not a few.

- ☐ **Watch the Calendar:** Before scheduling meetings and special events, make sure it's not a holiday. Remember that holidays like Hanukkah and Ramadan occur at different times each year, and be aware of holidays when scheduling patient appointments.

- ☐ **Let them eat cake:** Think of *everyone* when planning holiday parties and snacks. Send a note/email to find out about your colleagues' dietary needs and be mindful of the significance of religious dietary restrictions. Your colleagues are the best source of information about their needs.

- ☐ **Brown Bag It:** Find community members and guest speakers who can talk about different traditions. Invite co-workers to share what they do in December.

- ☐ **Winter Carnival:** Conduct several activities to celebrate different seasons or holidays—so that everyone at work can rotate or opt out without feeling awkward.

- ☐ **Learn New Phrases:** Learn about the different December holidays, their practices, and significance. Honor the differences with appropriate greetings for your colleagues and patients.

- ☐ **Bag or Box:** Think outside the box. Try a Grab Bag instead of a "Secret Santa." Gift giving is not specific to the holiday season. Consider doing a charity project together outside the office.

ADDENDUM: CHECKLISTS, TOOLS, & ORGANIZATIONAL RESOURCES

NAVIGATING THE DECEMBER DILEMMA: FIVE TO KNOW

Keep copies of this in an accessible location.

Hanukkah: Hanukkah, also known as the Festival of Lights or Festival of Rededication, is an eight-day Jewish holiday that starts on the 25th day of Kislev, which may be in December, late November, or, more rarely, early January. The festival is observed in Jewish homes by lighting candles on each of the festival's eight nights, one on the first night, two on the second night, and so on. Prayers are recited during this ritual. In some families, Hanukkah also includes gift-giving.

Christmas Day: Christmas is a holiday celebrating the birth of Jesus, the central figure of Christianity. Aspects of the celebration may include gift-giving, Christmas trees, church attendance, the Father Christmas/Santa Claus myth, and family gatherings. Most Western churches (e.g., the Protestant and Roman Catholic traditions) observe the holiday on December 25, while most Eastern Orthodox Churches celebrate on January 7.

The one exception is Jehovah's Witnesses, who, although Christian, do not celebrate Christmas, believing that it has pagan roots (along with other holidays like Easter and Thanksgiving).

Kwanzaa: Kwanzaa (or Kwaanza) is a week-long secular holiday honoring African-American heritage and community, celebrated almost exclusively by African-Americans. It is observed from December 26 to January 1.

Kwanzaa consists of seven days of celebration, featuring activities such as candle-lighting, drumming, the pouring of libations, and culminates in a feast and gift-giving. It was founded by controversial black nationalist Ron Karenga in 1966 as a way to foster African-American unity and culture.

Bodhi Day: Bodhi Day is usually observed on December 8, or the Sunday immediately preceding. This is the date, according to Mahayana Buddhist tradition, of Siddhartha Gautama (the historical Buddha)'s Enlightenment and the beginning of his Buddhist teachings.

Bodhi Day is usually observed with prayer and meditation.

Ramadan: For more than a billion Muslims around the world—including the approximately 6 million in North America—Ramadan is a month of prayer, fasting, and charity. Muslims believe that during the month of Ramadan, Allah revealed the first verses of the Qur'an, the holy book of Islam.

ADDENDUM: CHECKLISTS, TOOLS, & ORGANIZATIONAL RESOURCES

3

Working with Family, Friends and Other Caregivers: Organizational Resources

In many cases, especially with the elderly, young, or patients with long-term or degenerative conditions, practitioners work closely with other caregivers like family members, friends, visiting or live-in nurses, or other allied health professionals. These individuals can be tremendous assets in helping a patient get all of his or her religious needs met. (See the main text of Working with Family, Friends and Other Caregivers for more detailed information.)

When working with family, friends and other caregivers, there are three broad issues to think through:

1. Does the patient have religious needs that s/he will not be able to attend to him or herself?

2. In what ways can non-physician caregivers be most helpful in getting those religious needs met?

3. What do these other caregivers need to know about the patient's religious background and needs?

Thinking through each of these while planning a patient's discharge, home care or long-term hospital stay can help the practitioner create an effective and comprehensive team.

When working with a patient requiring family, friends or other caregivers, use the chart below to organize these relationships. Lay out what each caregiver's responsibilities and specific relationships to the patient are and use this information to think through how these caregivers might be of assistance with religious needs; this will inform what the caregivers need to know about the patient's religious beliefs and practices.

Chart on following page

ADDENDUM: CHECKLISTS, TOOLS, & ORGANIZATIONAL RESOURCES

CHART: Working with Family, Friends and Other Caregivers Tracking Sheet

Patient's Name _____   Supervising Physician _____

Caregiver's Name	Role/Relationship	Specific Responsibilities	Assistance with Religious Needs?	Contact Information

ADDENDUM: CHECKLISTS, TOOLS, & ORGANIZATIONAL RESOURCES

4
....
Pastoral Care: Organizational Resources

Understanding the role pastoral care professionals can play on the health care team is just the first step—the second is knowing who your chaplains are and where to find them.

If your office or facility has an intranet, consider making this chart available there for viewing and updating so that all staff members can easily access the information. This will help ensure that all staff members have the same knowledge base. Otherwise, keep this chart in a centralized location, such as a main desk or nurses' station. Make sure staff knows where the document sits so they can consult or update it with ease. To increase its utility, use this chart along with the tracking sheet for working with diverse communities; they will often intersect with one another.

In some instances—especially for those practitioners working in group practices or smaller facilities—there may be no on-site pastoral care professional(s). In that case, you may want to establish relationships with the pastoral care department of a larger facility with which you are affiliated, or with community religious leaders who may be useful resources.

It is also important to note whether or not a chaplain or community clergyperson has interfaith training and is able to work respectfully and effectively with patients from a variety of religious backgrounds; community clergy in particular are likely not equipped to do this. Where you have this information, include it in the chart to ensure that the clergyperson you call in can actually help you with your particular issue or patient.

Chart on following page

ADDENDUM: CHECKLISTS, TOOLS, & ORGANIZATIONAL RESOURCES

CHART: Chaplain & Clergy Contact Sheet

Name	Denominational or Church Affiliation	Contact Information	Interfaith?

ADDENDUM: CHECKLISTS, TOOLS, & ORGANIZATIONAL RESOURCES

5
....
Special Community Needs: Organizational Resources

Use the chart on the following page to keep track of the communities you serve (e.g., Russian Jewish, Thai Buddhist, etc.); where they are located and what particular facilities serve them (e.g., group practices or neighborhood clinics); what particular issues or barriers to health care they face, along with any responses or ideas your facility has had for dealing with them; the internal resources available to you for dealing with those issues (e.g., an employee who is a member of that community, journal articles or studies focused on providing culturally competent care for that community); and your external contacts — the people you can call on when an issue is beyond the capacity of your internal resources to address such as a chaplain, community leader or clergyperson.

 If your office or facility has an intranet, consider making this document available there for viewing and updating so that all staff members can easily access the information and share what they've learned about a particular community. This will help ensure that all staff members have the same knowledge base, and will create a living document to track your facility's efforts and suggest communities needing additional outreach.

 Otherwise, keep this chart at a centralized location such as a main desk or nurses' station. Make sure staff knows where it sits so that they can consult or update it with ease. To increase its utility, use this chart along with the tracking sheet for chaplains and community clergy contacts. They will often be good contacts for getting questions answered, or will be able to direct you to other resources.

 Be proactive and fill out this resource even if you don't think there are any access issues with the communities you serve; it will help you keep track of your diverse patient population.

Chart on following page

ADDENDUM: CHECKLISTS, TOOLS, & ORGANIZATIONAL RESOURCES

CHART: Special Community Needs Tracking Sheet

Community	Locations	Resources	Issues Noted / Responses	Contacts

NOTES

NOTES

NOTES

NOTES

NOTES

NOTES

NOTES

NOTES

NOTES